AIR FRYER COOKBOOK
Weight loss recipes

Sophia Moody

Copyright © 2021 Sophia Moody

All right deserved.

AIR FRYER COOKBOOK 1
Weight loss recipes 1
Sophia Moody 1

INTRODUCTION 8
What is an air fryer? 9
How an air fryer works 10
Advantages and disadvantages of a hot air fryer 12

BREAKFAST RECIPES 15
Breakfast wraps from the air fryer 15
Chocolate banana calzone from the hot air fryer 17
Fitness bread from the hot air fryer 19
Breakfast muffins from the air fryer 21
Rabas in the hot air fryer 23
Breaded Prawns in The Hot Air Fryer 24
A Bread Roll and An Egg 26
Poached eggs from the air fryer 28
Cucumber bread 30
Air Fryer Breakfast Sausage 31
Tomato and balsamic buns 33
Hawaii toast from the air fryer 35
Chocolate banana spread 37

SEAFOOD RECIPES AND FISH 39
Crispy fish roll from the air fryer 39
Fish fillet with herbs wrapped in baking paper from the hot air fryer 41
Fish lasagne with beetroot from the hot air fryer 43
Crunchy salmon cubes from the hot air fryer 46
Florentine fish from the air fryer 48
Homemade fish fingers from the hot air fryer 50
Fish fillet with herbs wrapped in baking paper from the hot air fryer 52
Salmon with fennel and orange from the air fryer 54
Salmon with Baked Potatoes 56
Tuna spread 58
Philadelphia lemon dumplings 59
Fast fish burger 61
Pickled salmon trout sandwich 63
Cottage fish spread 64
Fried wild salmon fillet 65

Salmon spread with curd cheese 66
Smoked trout spread 67
Shrimp soup with green asparagus 69

POULTRY RECIPES 71

Spicy chicken drumsticks with grill marinade from the hot air fryer 71
Mediterranean chicken nuggets from the hot air fryer 73
Chicken nuggets from the air fryer 75
Filled pita with turkey and vegetables from the hot air fryer 77
Chicken curry skewers from the hot air fryer 79
Fried chicken salad from the hot air fryer 81
Chicken breast on grilled vegetables from the air fryer 83
Air Fryer BBQ Wings 86
Ham-wrapped turkey 88
Jamaican jerk turkey 89
Turkey in the port wine bath 91
Tuna with a fruity cucumber salad 92

BEEF RECIPES 94

Meat skewers with letscho from the air fryer 94
Frittata with corn, paprika and grilled turkey cubes 96
Express beef roulades in a caper cream sauce 98
Beef roulades from the air fryer 100
Beef steak with onion vegetables 102
Corned beef sandwich 104
Grilled beef steak 106
Sliced beef 108
Wok vegetables with meat 110
Beef and green beans salad 112
Meatballs with green salad 114
Hearty turnip and carrot stew with beef 116
Smart beef goulash basic recipe 119
Meat vegetable strudel 121
Roast steak perfectly 123

PORK RECIPES 124

Roast pork from the air fryer 124
Spare ribs from the air fryer 127
Pork rack fried in water 129
Fried pork rack 131
Stuffed meat roll 132
Pork stew 134
Caribbean style spare ribs 136
Spare ribs the hell of a way 138
Pork in cider batter 140

Pork medallions...142
Baked Hawaiian schnitzel 144
Pork steaks with chanterelles 146
Fried pork rack 148
Boneless drumstick in a simple oven..149

VEGETABLE RECIPES 151
Mini peppers with goat cheese from the hot air fryer 151
Potato and vegetable chips from the hot air fryer......................153
Potato gratin with wild garlic..155
Asparagus lasagna from the hot air fryer 157
Pumpkin fritters from the air fryer...159
Spinach strudel from the hot air fryer...161
Baked vegetables from the air fryer...163
Cooked oven vegetables from the air fryer 165
Crispy spring rolls from the hot air fryer....................................167
Red-white-red casserole from the air fryer 169
Sweet potato fries from the air fryer..171
Spicy puff pastry roses from the hot air fryer 172
Vegetable nuggets from the air fryer 174
Chanterelle goulash from the hot air fryer.................................176
Light potato and zucchini patties from the hot air fryer...........178
Vegetable and oat patties from the hot air fryer........................180
Zucchini chips from the air fryer 182
Zucchini and feta casserole from the hot air fryer 184
Corn skewers from the air fryer...186

Side Dish..187
Air Fryer corn on The Cob..187
Air Fryer Potato Latkes 189
Sampan Copycat: Air Fried Brussels Sprouts..............................191
Air-Fried Pickles with Chipotle Dipping Sauce............................193
Air Fryer Avocado Fries + Sriracha Ketchup 195
Air Fryer Buffalo Turkey Meatball 197
Raclette In the Air fryer 200
Rack of Lamb with Herb Crust from The Air fryer 202
Spicy Carrots from The Air fryer...205
COQ Au Vin from The Air fryer..207
Air Fryer Corn on The Cob...209
Egg Salad..211
Potato and rocket salad...213
Potato and celery puree 215
Semolina dumplings 216
Croquettes from the air fryer...218

    Pumpkin wedges from the air fryer 219
    Corn skewers from the air fryer... 220

DESSERT, SWEETS AND SNACKS 222
    Fried Bananas S'mores.. 222
    Air fryer Apple Pie.. 224
    Roasted Apples in Jocca Oil-Free Fryer 227
    Baked Apple from The Air fryer 229
    Crispy baked apple with rum and raisins 230
    Strawberry muffins 232
    Plantain Chips.. 234
    Bruschette with tomato topping 235
    Sandwich cake 236
    Baked tuna breads 237
    Fried onion 238
    Minced patties... 239
    Breaded zucchini 241
    Air Fryer Sweet Potato Tots 242
    Air Fryer Banana Bread 244
    Air Fryer Avocado Fries 246
    Air Fryer Southern Style Catfish With Green Beans............................ 251
    Air Fryer Strawberry Pop Tarts 254

Air Fryer Empanadas...*256*
    Air-Fried Peach Hand Pies 259
    Mexican-Style Air-Fried Corn.. 261

Air-Fried Whole-Wheat Pita Pizzas *263*

Air-Fried Coconut Shrimp *265*
    Air-Fried Corn Dog Bites... 268
    Crispy Toasted Sesame Tofu.. 271
    Air-Fried Beet Chips 274
    Air Fryer Veggie Quesadillas... 275
    Air-Fried Breakfast Bombs.. 278
    Air-Fried Curry Chickpeas... 281
    Air Fryer "Everything Bagel" Kale Chips 283
    Air Fry These Shrimp Spring Rolls With Sweet Chili Sauce 285
    Spicy Zucchini Slices... 288
    Cheddar Portobello Mushrooms 290
    Salty Lemon Artichokes.. 292
    Cheddar Potato Gratin 294
    Breaded Air Fried Shrimp with Bang-Bang Sauce 296
    Shrimp Egg Rolls 298
    Chocolate Almond Butter Brownie.. 300

Parmesan Sweet Potato Casserole 302
Asparagus & Parmesan 304

INTRODUCTION

In the constant boom of technology, new things always come to our home that promise to simplify or improve our lives. This time it was the turn of the air fryer (Air fryer), there is an open debate between if this appliance Is arriving to improve our health. It is only a job well done on marketing.

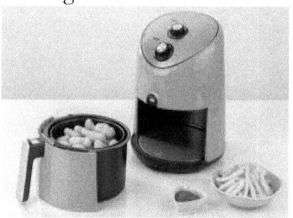

An air fryer's main premise is that we do not need to immerse our food for an extended period in oil to obtain that incredible flavor and crunchy texture. With only half a tablespoon of oil, it is enough for 10 or 15 minutes to get the same delicious results.

Most of the foods prepared within this cooking device do not require oil at all, only hot air. Based on Rapid Air technology, air fryers blow superheated air to cook foods that would traditionally be fried in oil.

To clarify this controversial debate, we must first understand how an air fryer works, different types, and how to use it.

What is an air fryer?

Vegetables, red and white meats, fish, eggs and shellfish, young and old can hardly resist this temptation.

However, overconsumption of deep-fried foods is not healthy. Frying is high in saturated fat, high in calories, and difficult to digest. And no self-respecting nutritionist or dietician would be able to say they do not use this sort of preparation for a healthy diet.

Some appliances make up for the use of fats and fatty oils, but these appliances also use heat to fry food.

These are the "air fryers" that imitate traditional deep fat fryers, but with more healthy and ecologically sound results.

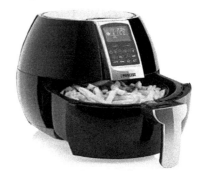

An advantage is that these fryers can quickly cut off the smell of fried food even for days and days.

Air fryers do not fry oil, just heated air. Even if you do not have a microwave oven, you can use a pan because hot air cooks. In this space, the air flows quickly and high temperatures are reached, making cooking easy.

How an air fryer works

We have seen that the hot air fryer works thanks to a special cooking chamber where the air circulates so fast that it reaches very high temperatures.

Thanks to the high temperatures, the oil reaches a degree of heat suitable for frying food and a simple heat carrier since it is the hot air that ensures uniform cooking.

Similarly, to a traditional deep fryer, with the air fryer, you do not need to immerse the food in a large amount of frying oil and you do not need to turn the food stuffy.

Foods are surrounded by very hot air and become crunchy on the outside and soft on the inside in a matter of minutes. Furthermore, this technique is useful in keeping the properties of food intact.

The heating chamber's hot air can reach temperatures close to 200 °. This makes air fryers extremely useful appliances and very energy-intensive: the average electrical consumption ranges from 800 to 2,000 watts. However, the economic return (less oil used) and health benefits should not be underestimated.

Advantages and disadvantages of a hot air fryer

The hot air fryer is spreading rapidly in many households and offers a wide range of options. In addition to the many advantages, there are also some disadvantages associated with such a device. We will now go into this in the following text. The great advantage of preparing food in the hot air fryer is that the food is lower in fat and healthier than the food from the classic deep fryer. The dishes are not deep-fried here, but rather baked in hot air until they are crispy.

Even more advantages of a hot air fryer

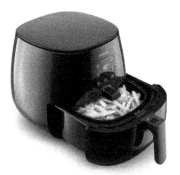

Another advantage of a hot air fryer is that the original taste of the food is preserved. Because little or no oil is used, the foods used retain their natural taste and appearance.

Also, the food is prepared faster, which saves electricity. Thanks to the gentle preparation, more vitamins are retained in the food than with a conventional deep fryer.

Also, the options for using a hot air fryer are much more diverse. In such a device, you can not only deep-fry food but also bake pizza, rolls, cakes, or bread . You can also cook stews, steam fish or meat or prepare gratins in a hot air fryer.

Furthermore, it is pleasant that a hot air fryer does not cause the typical frying smell. Such a device is very easy to handle and can be cleaned quickly and easily after use.

But there are also disadvantages

However, there are also some disadvantages associated with using a hot air fryer. On the one hand, dishes such as French fries or nuggets are not as crispy as they are in the classic deep fryer. On the other hand, it is also the case that the juiciness can decrease. This means that some dishes can dry out faster due to the hot air and are no longer quite juicy.

Also, the preparation time with a hot air fryer is shortened due to the shorter preheating time, but the actual cooking process is longer than a conventional device.

BREAKFAST RECIPES

Breakfast wraps from the air fryer

- Cooking time 5 to 15 min
- Servings: 2

Ingredients

- 2 pc tortillas (bought ready)
- 2 eggs
- 3 tbsp cheese (of your choice, grated)
- 2 tbsp yoghurt
- 2 slices of bacon
- 1 tomato
- 4 pcs. Mushrooms
- 2 tbsp chives (fresh, cut into fine pieces)
- Iceberg lettuce
- salt
- pepper

Preparation

1. Made super-fast in the morning, thanks to the rapid temperature heating in the Airfryer!
2. For the Breakfast Wraps, fry the bacon in the Airfryer hot air fryer at 180 ° C and lift it out again. Beat the eggs, season with salt and pepper and pour into the Airfryer pan. Let it set until creamy at 170 ° C, stirring constantly. Cut the tomato and mushrooms into large pieces. Mix the yoghurt and chives, season with salt and pepper.
3. Briefly warm up the tortillas in the Airfryer.
4. Spread the yoghurt cream on the warm tortillas, place the egg dish, bacon, tomatoes and mushrooms, sprinkle with cheese and top with some lettuce leaves.
5. Roll up the wraps and enjoy!
6. Perfect served with an iceberg lettuce and the remaining yogurt sauce!

Chocolate banana calzone from the hot air fryer

- Cooking time 15 to 30 min
- Servings: 4

Ingredients

- 1 pkg of pizza dough
- 2 bananas
- 4 tbsp nougat cream
- 2 tbsp hazelnuts (ground)
- 200 ml whipped cream (whipped)

Preparation

1. For the chocolate and banana calzone, first roll out the pizza dough and cut out 4 circles about 15 cm in diameter. Spread 1 tablespoon of nougat cream in the middle, leaving about 1 cm free at the edge.

2. Peel the bananas and cut into thin slices. Place on top of the nougat cream. Scatter the hazelnuts on top.
3. Fold the dough circles together and press the edges firmly into place. Bake in the Airfryer hot air fryer at 200 ° C for about 10 minutes.
4. To serve, whip the whipped cream until stiff and use it to serve the chocolate and banana calzone.

Fitness bread from the hot air fryer

- Cooking time More than 60 min
- Servings: 4

Ingredients

- 150 g whole wheat flour
- 150 g wholemeal rye flour
- 1 tbsp agave syrup
- 25 g germ
- 1 tbsp flaxseed oil
- 1 teaspoon salt
- 40 g walnuts
- 35 g pumpkin seeds
- 50 g dried fruit (of your choice)
- Water (for brushing)

Preparation

1. For the fitness bread, sieve rye flour and wheat flour together and season with salt. Dissolve the yeast in lukewarm water and stir in agave syrup. Mix with the flour, add

the oil and knead everything into a smooth dough.
2. Cover and let the dough rise in a warm place for about 30 minutes.
3. In the meantime, coarsely chop the nuts and kernels and cut the dried fruit into small pieces.
4. The dough has increased in volume during the resting phase. Now quickly knead in the nuts, kernels and fruit and distribute well.
5. Pour the batter directly into the Airfryer hot air fryer's baking pan or shape it into a loaf and place on baking paper in the grid insert, cover and let rise for another 15 minutes.
6. Bake the bread dough in the Airfryer hot air fryer at 200 ° C for 5 minutes. Then reduce the temperature to 180 ° C and bake for another 55 minutes. This will make the crust even crisper.
7. The fitness bread from time to time with a little water and sprinkle makes the crust nice shine.

Breakfast muffins from the air fryer

- Cooking time 30 to 60 min
- Servings: 4

Ingredients

- 4 slice (s) of toast bread
- 4 slices of bacon
- Butter (liquid)
- 4 eggs
- salt
- Pepper (from the mill)

Preparation

1. First, the breakfast muffins from the hot air fryer flatten the toast and cut out as large a circle as possible from each slice. Cut in the middle.
2. Skip the bacon. But it shouldn't get too crispy so that it can still be bent.
3. Grease muffin moulds (made of silicone for the Airfryer) and line them with 2

semicircles of toast. There should be no hole left. Possibly help with the sections. Place a slice of bacon in each and let an egg run in. Salt and pepper.
4. The breakfast muffins for 15 minutes at 190 ° C in about Airfryer bake.

Rabas in the hot air fryer

- Cooking time 30 to 60 min
- Servings: 4

Ingredients

- 16 rabies
- 1 egg
- Bread crumbs
- Condiments: salt, pepper, sweet paprika

Preparation

1. In my case, they were frozen, so I put them in hot water, and they boil for 2 minutes.
2. Remove and dry well.
3. Beat the egg and season to taste. I put salt, pepper, and sweet paprika — place in the egg.
4. Spray with fritolin and place 5 more minutes at 200 degrees.

Breaded Prawns in The Hot Air Fryer

- Cooking time 10 to 20 min
- Servings: 4

Ingredients

- 9 raw prawns
- 1 egg
- Bread crumbs
- Condiments: salt, pepper, and sweet paprika

Preparation

1. As the prawns were clean but raw and frozen, I put them in water and let them boil for 2 minutes.
2. Remove from water and dry with absorbent paper.
3. Beat the egg and season to taste. In my case, as my daughter eats, I did not put anything spicy. Place them on a stick of

brochettes and brush with the beaten egg. Leave in the egg until breading.
4. Bread with breadcrumbs. Brush again with egg and breading again.
5. Place in the fryer strainer. Cook 5 minutes at 160 degrees. Remove
6. Spray with fritolin or brush with oil. Place 5 more minutes in the fryer at 200 degrees. Ready to enjoy them.

A Bread Roll and An Egg

- Cooking time 15 to 30 min
- Servings: 4

Ingredients

- 4 whole-grain bread rolls
- 4 eggs
- 40g spring onions
- 8 slices bacon
- 50gn butter
- 80g cheese
- Salt pepper

Preparation

1. Cut in the rolls above and hollow out with the help of a spoon. Chop the spring onions, mix with the cheese and season a bit.
2. Spread buns with butter and cover with bacon, separate eggs. Add the egg whites

to the spring onion and cheese and fill them with a spoon in the bread. Put the egg yolk on top.
3. Bake the rolls at 160 ° C for 10-12 minutes in the baking tray of the Airfryer. Tip: With a flake butter, you can refine the buns again. To test whether your buns are even, you can look up with the wooden skewers trick. If it sticks, give the bun for another minute.

Poached eggs from the air fryer

- Cooking time 30 min
- Servings: 2

Ingredients

- 2 Owner
- Avocado
- 1 clove of garlic
- 3-6 Cherrytomaten
- 1L boiling water
- 50ml vinegar
- 1-2 EL   Sriracha Sauce
- Parsley, salt & pepper

Preparation

1. To poach the eggs, pour 1l boiling water into the air fryer's baking mould and add the vinegar. Then carefully insert the eggs into the liquid and if necessary, hold them

together with a spoon. Cook for 3-5 minutes in the Airfryer at 200 ° C.
2. For the spread, chop an avocado, garlic, and tomatoes. Mix with a little Sriracha sauce, olive oil and a little salt. Serve everything on a slice of toasted bread and garnish with parsley and lemon zest.

Cucumber bread

- Cooking time 5 to 15 min
- Servings: 1

Ingredients

- 1 slice (s) of farmhouse bread
- butter
- 1/4 cucumber
- 1 pinch of salt
- 1 pinch of pepper
- 1 tbsp dill (chopped)
- 2 tbsp sour cream

Preparation

1. Spread a thin layer of butter on the farmer's bread.
2. Peel the cucumber and cut into slices. Spread on the bread. Sprinkle with salt and pepper.
3. Chop the dill, pour over it and garnish with sour cream.

Air Fryer Breakfast Sausage

- Cooking time 5 to 15 min
- Servings: 8

Ingredients

- 1pound ground pork
- 1 pound ground turkey
- 2 teaspoons fennel seeds
- 2 teaspoons dried sage rubbed
- 2 teaspoons garlic powder
- 1 teaspoon of paprika
- 1 teaspoon of sea salt
- 1 teaspoon dried thyme
- 1 tablespoon real maple syrup

Preparation

1. Start by mixing the pork and turkey in a large bowl. In a small bowl, mix the remaining ingredients: fennel, sage, garlic powder, paprika, salt, and thyme. Pour

spices into the meat and continue mixing until the spices are fully incorporated.
2. Scoop into balls (about 2-3 tablespoons of meat), and flatten into patties. Place inside the fryer, you will probably have to do this in 2 batches.
3. Set the temperature to 370 degrees and cook for 10 minutes. Remove from the fryer and repeat with the remaining sausage.

Tomato and balsamic buns

- Preparation: 15 mins
- Cooking time 30mins
- Servings 4

Ingredients

- 1 g pepper
- 1 g salt
- 1 g of oregano
- 360 g black bread
- 120 g mozzarella
- 150 g tomatoes
- 30 g balsamic vinegar

Preparation

1. For the tomato and balsamic bun, first sprinkle the bread slices with a little balsamic vinegar.

2. Then cover with tomato slices and mozzarella and sprinkle with salt, pepper and oregano.
3. Then put it in the oven for about 10 minutes at 180 degrees Celsius until the cheese has melted. A mixed leaf salad goes best with the tomato and balsamic bun.

Hawaii toast from the air fryer

- Preparation: 15 mins
- Cooking time 30mins
- Servings 2

Ingredients

- 4 slice (s) of toast
- 120 g ham
- 100 g pineapple (diced)
- Butter (for brushing)
- salt
- pepper
- 100 g cheese

Preparation

1. First toast and butter the bread slices.
2. Top with ham and pineapple and season with salt and pepper to taste. Put the cheese on top.

3. Briefly gratin ate the Hawaii toast in the hot air fryer.
4. Then arrange and serve.

Chocolate banana spread

- Preparation: 15 minutes
- Servings 4

Ingredients

- 50 g dark chocolate
- 250 g lactose-free quark (20% fat)
- 2 tbsp oat drink (oat milk)
- 1 banana
- 4 slices oat bread

Preparation

1. Finely grate the dark chocolate. Set aside about 1 tbsp of the rasp.
2. Mix the quark with the oat drink until smooth. Fold in the chocolate flakes.
3. Peel the banana and cut it diagonally into slices.
4. Spread the chocolate quark on the bread, place the banana slices on top and

sprinkle with the remaining chocolate shavings.

SEAFOOD RECIPES AND FISH

Crispy fish roll from the air fryer

- Cooking time 15 to 30 min
- Servings: 2

Ingredients

- 150 g fish fillets (white, skinless, chopped)
- 1 pinch of salt
- pepper
- 1 tbsp lemon juice (freshly squeezed)
- 3-4 spring roll leaves (from the Asian store)
- Egg white (for gluing the rolls)
- Egg yolk (for brushing the rolls)
- 1 tbsp butter (liquid)

Preparation

1. For the crispy fish roll, wash the fish fillet, pat dry and chop finely. Then season the

fish with salt, pepper and lemon juice and mix everything thoroughly.
2. Spread the spring roll dough on the work surface. Place the marinated fish in a line in the middle of the leaves.
3. Brush the edges of the pastry thinly with egg white. Fold in the spring roll leaves on the left and right, roll up tightly and then brush the outside with the egg yolk and butter mixture on both sides.
4. Bake the fish rolls in the hot air fryer for 11–13 minutes at 180 ° C. The crispy fish role inflicts arbitrary and serve.

Fish fillet with herbs wrapped in baking paper from the hot air fryer

- Cooking time 15 to 30 min

Ingredients

- 50 g cherry tomatoes
- 1/2 clove (s) garlic (diced)
- 1/4 lemon (thinly sliced)
- 150 g fish fillets (skinless)
- pinch of sea salt
- 1 pinch of pepper
- 50 g peas
- 1 pinch of saffron threads
- 20 ml white wine
- tbsp olive oil
- 1 sprig (s) of thyme (plucked)
- Chervil (chopped)

Preparation

1. For the fish fillet with herbs in baking paper, wash the cherry tomatoes and cut

in half, peel the garlic and press down with the knife. Wash the lemon with hot water, dry it and then cut it into thin slices.
2. Wash the fish fillets, pat dry and season with sea salt and pepper.
3. Cut a large sheet of parchment paper (if the fish is on it, you must still tie the ends of the sheet).
4. Distribute all ingredients in portions on the sheet of baking paper, add the peas and saffron. Drizzle with wine and olive oil, season well with sea salt and pepper and refine with the herbs.
5. Fold up the sheets of paper and tie tightly with kitchen thread. The fish fillet with herbs in the baking paper jacket in the Airfryer and cook for 12-15 minutes at 200 ° C.
6. When the packet is opened, the filling smells wonderfully aromatic.

Fish lasagne with beetroot from the hot air fryer

- Cooking time 30 to 60 min
- Servings: 2

Ingredients

- 300 g fish fillets (from freshwater fish)
- 300 g lasagne sheets
- 150 g beets (peeled)
- 250 ml milk
- 25 g butter
- 30 grams of flour
- salt
- Pepper (from the mill)
- Nutmeg (grated)
- 1/2 lemon
- Dill (fresh)
- 50 g parmesan (grated)
- olive oil

Preparation

1. For the fish lasagne with beetroot, bring a saucepan with approx. 3 liters of water to the boil. Salt well and cook the lasagne sheets in it for about 5-6 minutes, stirring frequently to prevent them from sticking together.
2. Remove from the water, drain well and put a little olive oil on a piece of baking paper.
3. Heat the milk with salt and pepper. Melt the butter in a small saucepan, let it foam and quickly stir the flour in it until smooth. Pour in the hot milk, stirring constantly, and simmer for about 2 minutes. Stir constantly. Finally, season with grated lemon zest and nutmeg, season to taste.
4. Slice the beetroot into thin slices, season with salt and let steep for about 5 minutes.
5. Remove skin and bones from the fish fillets, cut in half flat if necessary. Season with salt and lemon juice.
6. Spread a little béchamel sauce on the baking pan. Lay alternately layers of

lasagna dough sheets, sauce, fish fillets, some fresh dill and beetroot in the mold. Repeat 2-3 times, finally spread the parmesan on top.
7. Bake in the hot air fryer at 160 ° C for about 20-25 minutes.
8. Let the fish lasagne with beetroot cool down a little before serving!

Crunchy salmon cubes from the hot air fryer

- Cooking time 15 to 30 min
- Servings: 4

Ingredients

- 200 g salmon fillet (skinless and bones)
- some flour
- 1 egg
- 100 g corn flakes (crumbled)
- 1 tuber (s) of fennel
- 1 lemon
- 1 pinch of sugar
- some sprinkles of balsamic vinegar
- olive oil
- salt
- pepper

Preparation

1. For crispy salmon cubes from the hot air fryer, first cut the salmon fillet into approx. 3 x 3 cm cubes and season with a little lemon juice, salt and pepper. Bread in flour, beaten egg and corn flakes. Bake in the Philips Airfryer hot air fryer at 190 ° C for approx. 6-8 minutes.
2. Wash the fennel, cut in half and remove the stalk. Then cut or slice into fine strips. Mix with salt, pepper, lemon juice and olive oil, season to taste and leave to marinate for about 10 minutes.
3. Serve crispy salmon cubes from the hot air fryer with the fennel and drizzle with some balsamic vinegar.

Florentine fish from the air fryer

- Cooking time 15 to 30 min
- Servings: 1

Ingredients

- 130 g spinach leaves (frozen)
- 1 clove (s) of garlic
- salt
- pepper
- nutmeg
- 130 g fish fillets (polar cod, salmon, char, ..)
- Lemon juice
- 130 g roasted potatoes (or oven-roasted rabbits)
- 50 g cheese (grated, Cheddar, Gouda, ...)

Preparation

1. For the Florentine-style fish, thaw spinach leaves, cut into small pieces and allow to thaw completely. Mix the spinach with a

finely chopped clove of garlic, salt, pepper, and grated nutmeg and pour into the air fryer's casserole dish.
2. Rub the fish fillets on both sides with salt and a little lemon juice and place them next to each other on the bed of spinach leaves. Spread the roasted potatoes on top and cover everything with the grated cheese.
3. Bake at 180 °C for 15 minutes until the surface is brown and serve.

Homemade fish fingers from the hot air fryer

- Cooking time 15 to 30 min
- Servings: 4

Ingredients

- 500 g halibut (or other fish with firm meat)
- salt
- pepper
- 1-2 eggs
- Flour
- Breadcrumbs
- Oil

Preparation

1. For the homemade fish fingers from the hot air fryer, first wash, dry, salt and pepper the fish. Cut into sticks.

2. Set up a breading line: First prepare a plate with flour, then with the beaten eggs and finally with breadcrumbs.
3. Turn the fish strips one after the other in the flour, egg and breadcrumbs.
4. Bake in the air fryer with a little oil at 180 ° C for about 7-10 minutes.
5. The fish fingers from the air fryer serve immediately.

Fish fillet with herbs wrapped in baking paper from the hot air fryer

- Cooking time 5 to 15 min
- Servings: 1

Ingredient

- 50 g cherry tomatoes
- 1/2 clove (s) garlic (diced)
- 1/4 lemon (thinly sliced)
- 150 g fish fillets (skinless)
- 1 pinch of sea salt
- 1 pinch of pepper
- 50 g peas
- 1 pinch of saffron threads
- 20 ml white wine
    - tbsp olive oil
- 1 sprig (s) of thyme (plucked)
- Chervil (chopped)

Preparation

1. For the fish fillet with herbs in baking paper, wash the cherry tomatoes and cut in half, peel the garlic and press down with the knife. Wash the lemon with hot water, dry it and then cut it into thin slices.
2. Wash the fish fillets, pat dry and season with sea salt and pepper.
3. Cut a large sheet of parchment paper (if the fish is on it, you must still tie the ends of the sheet).
4. Distribute all ingredients in portions on the sheet of baking paper, add the peas and saffron. Drizzle with wine and olive oil, season well with sea salt and pepper and refine with the herbs.
5. Fold up the sheets of paper and tie tightly with kitchen thread. The fish fillet with herbs in baking paper jacket in the Airfryer and cook for 12-15 minutes at 200 ° C.
6. When the packet is opened, the filling smells wonderfully aromatic.

Salmon with fennel and orange from the air fryer

- Preparation time 5mins
- Cooking time 30mins
- Servings 2

Ingredients

- 3 Tablespoons olive oil
- 1 orange
- 300g salmon
- 1 fennel
- 1 Bunch dill
- Salt pepper

Preparation

1. Cut the orange and fennel into even slices and season with a dash of olive oil and some salt and pepper. Bake at 160 ° C for 10 minutes.

2. Now put the bunch dill on the fennel and the oranges and embed the salmon on it. Season again with a little salt, pepper, and olive oil and grate some orange peel on the fish. Bake again for 10 minutes at 160 ° C in the Airfryer and ready!

Salmon with Baked Potatoes

- Preparation time: 50 min
- servings 4

Ingredients

- 1 kg smaller potatoes
- 3 blue onions
- 4 salmon fillets with skin
- 2 tbsp butter
- 2 tbsp rapeseed oil
- iodized salt with fluoride
- pepper
- 1 tbsp harissa

Preparation

1. Peel the onions and cut into strips. Peel and halve the potatoes. Sauté the onions in the butter and place in a baking dish. Mix in Harissa.
2. Sauté the potatoes in the oil and spread over the onions, season everything with salt and pepper.

3. Put in the preheated oven and bake at 200 ° C for about 25-30 minutes. After 10 minutes pour in 50 ml of water. After 15-20 minutes, lightly salt the fish and place it on the potatoes with the skin facing upwards and finish cooking.

Tuna spread

- Prep time 30 min
- Servings 4

Ingredients

- 1 can (s) of tuna (in its juice, drained)
- 130 g sour cream
- 1 tbsp mayonnaise
- 1 tbsp capers
- 1 dash of lemon juice
- salt
- Pepper (from the mill)

Preparation

1. For the tuna spread, first drain the capers and chop them finely.
2. Mix all ingredients well to form a smooth tuna spread.

Philadelphia lemon dumplings

- preparation time 5mins
- cooking time 15mins
- servings 4

Ingredients

- 175 g Philadelphia double cream setting natural
- 20 g flour (handy)
- 1/2 lemon
- 1 pc egg
- 20 g butter (melted)
- A bit of salt
- 1 tbsp white breadcrumbs (fine)

Preparation

1. For the Philadelphia lemon dumplings, grate the zest of half a lemon and squeeze half a lemon.

2. Mix all ingredients and cut out dumplings with a wet tablespoon.
3. Put the dumplings in boiling water and let stand for about 3 minutes.

Fast fish burger

- Preparation time 5mins
- Cooking time 10mins
- Servings 2

Ingredients

- 2 fish patties
- some butter
- 2 slice (s) of cheese
- 2 sheets of Güner lettuce
- 4 tomato slices
- 2 burger buns
- tartare sauce
- Ketchup
- onion rings

Preparation

1. For the quick fish burger, fry the fish patties in the pan - at the end of the roasting time, melt a slice of cheese on each of the fish patties.

2. Spread the burger buns with tartar sauce and arrange the lettuce, tomato slices and onion rings on top.
3. Place a fish loaf (with cheese) on each burger bun (with tartare / lettuce/tomato / onion sauce) and top with ketchup.
4. Finish with the burger bun lid.

Pickled salmon trout sandwich

Ingredients

- Ciabatte (or white bread)
- 2 slices of salmon trout (graved)
- 1 tbsp cream cheese (natural)
- 1 teaspoon honey mustard dill sauce
- Lettuce leaves
- Cucumber slices

Preparation

1. For the sandwich with pickled salmon trout, cut the ciabatta bread in half, spread the lower half with cream cheese and cover with the lettuce leaves.
2. Place the salmon trout slices on top and brush with the honey and mustard sauce. Finish with cucumber slices and the top half of the bread.

Cottage fish spread

Ingredients

- 250 g cottage cheese
- 1/2 bunch of chives
- 1 can (s) of tuna (natural)
- salt
- pepper
- 1 squirt of lemon juice

Preparation

1. For the cottage fish spread, wash and finely chop the chives. Chop up the tuna. Mix the cottage cheese with the chives, tuna and lemon juice.
2. Season with salt and pepper.

Fried wild salmon fillet

Ingredients

- 60 days wild salmon fillet
- 8 dag butter
- salt
- pepper
- Chilli flakes

Preparation

1. For the roasted wild salmon fillet, salt and pepper the wild salmon fillets and sprinkle with a few chilli flakes. Heat the butter in a pan and fry the salmon fillets on both sides.
2. Arrange and serve.

Salmon spread with curd cheese

- preparation time 5mins
- cooking time 15mins
- servings 4

Ingredients

- 250 g curd cheese
- 200 g smoked salmon (finely chopped)
- 1/2 lemon (juice)
- salt
- pepper
- Herbs (as desired)

Preparation

1. Finely chop the smoked salmon.
2. Mix the curd cheese, smoked salmon, lemon juice, herbs of your choice, salt and pepper together well.
3. Season again to taste and serve.

Smoked trout spread

- preparation time 10 mins
- cooking time 10 mins
- servings 4

Ingredients

- 1 cup of creme fraiche
- 3 eggs (hard-boiled)
- 2 trout (smoked)
- 3 tbsp herbs (chopped)
- pinch of pepper
- 1/2 cup of sour cream
- 1 squirt of lemon juice
- Salt

Preparation

1. For the smoked trout spread, peel the hard-boiled eggs cut them finely and place in a bowl. Chop the trout fillets and add.

2. Mix with creme fraiche and sour cream to make a spreadable fish spread. Finally, season with a splash of lemon juice and the chopped herbs.
3. Season to taste with salt and pepper and leave the smoked trout spread in the refrigerator for about 60 minutes.

Shrimp soup with green asparagus

- Preparation: 20 min
- servings 2

Ingredients

- 400 g green asparagus
- 1 tbsp oil
- 1 onion
- 1 clove of garlic
- 6 shrimp deveined ready to cook and peeled except for the tail segment
- 500 ml vegetable broth
- 1 tsp cornmeal
- 1 egg
- salt
- pepper from the mill
- soy sauce
- chives roll for garnish

Preparation

1. Peel and halve the lower third of the asparagus.
2. Peel and finely chop the onion and garlic. Sweat slowly with the asparagus in hot oil for approx. 5-6 minutes. Then add the prawns, fry them, dust with corn flour and deglaze with the broth. Bring to the boil and let simmer for about 1-2 minutes, then stir in the beaten egg and finally season with salt, pepper and soy sauce. Spread the soup on preheated plates and serve sprinkled with chives.

POULTRY RECIPES

Spicy chicken drumsticks with grill marinade from the hot air fryer

- Cooking time 30 to 60 min
- Servings: 4

Ingredients

- 1 clove (s) of garlic (crushed)
- 1/2 tbsp mustard
- 2 tsp sugar (brown)
- 1 teaspoon chilli powder
- Pepper (black, freshly ground)
- 1 tbsp olive oil
- 5 pieces of chicken lower legs

Preparation

1. For the spicy chicken drumsticks with grill marinade, mix the garlic with mustard, brown sugar, chilli powder, a pinch of salt and freshly ground pepper. Mix with the oil.
2. Rub the chicken thighs completely with the marinade and marinate for 20 minutes.
3. Put the chicken thighs in the basket and slide the basket into the air fryer. Set the timer for 10-12 minutes.
4. Fry the chicken thighs at 200 ° C until brown. Then reduce the temperature to 150 ° C and fry the chicken thighs for another 10 minutes until they are cooked through.
5. The spicy chicken leg with barbecue marinade with corn salad and baguette serve.

Mediterranean chicken nuggets from the hot air fryer

- Cooking time 30 to 60 min
- Servings: 4

Ingredients

- 2 slice (s) of white bread (old, in pieces)
- 1 tbsp paprika powder (hot)
- 1 tbsp olive oil
- 250 g chicken breast fillet (in pieces)
- 1 egg yolk
- 1 egg white
- 1 clove (s) of garlic (crushed)
- 2 teaspoons pesto (red)
- Pepper (freshly ground)
- 1 tbsp parsley (smooth, finely chopped)

Preparation

1. For Mediterranean chicken nuggets, grind the bread with the paprika powder in the

food processor to a crumbly mass; Stir in the olive oil. Put this mixture in a bowl.
2. Then puree the chicken breast fillet in the food processor and mix with the egg yolk, garlic, pesto and parsley. Season to taste with 1/2 teaspoon salt and a little pepper.
3. Beat the egg whites in a bowl. Shape the mixture into 10 balls and flatten it into oval nuggets.
4. Turn the nuggets first in the egg white and then in the breadcrumbs. The nuggets must be fully breaded.
5. Put five nuggets in the basket and slide the basket into the air fryer. Set the timer for 10-12 minutes. Fry the nuggets until golden brown at 200 ° C. Then fry the remaining nuggets.
6. Mediterranean chicken nuggets are best served with French fries and fresh salad.

Chicken nuggets from the air fryer

- Cooking time 15 to 30 min
- Servings: 4

Ingredients

- 500 g chicken fillet (skin and bone)
- 150 g flour (smooth)
- 2-3 eggs
- 50 ml whipped cream
- 200 g of breadcrumbs
- Salt
- 1 teaspoon sunflower oil

Preparation

1. Cut the chicken breast into bite-sized pieces.
2. Beat the eggs and whisk with cream and salt.
3. First turn the chicken pieces in flour, pull them through the eggs and finally bread them with the breadcrumbs.

4. Bake in the hot air fryer with a little oil at 180 °C for about 9-11 minutes until crispy.
5. Salt the chicken nuggets and serve with homemade fries, for example.

Filled pita with turkey and vegetables from the hot air fryer

- Cooking time 15 to 30 min
- Servings: 4

Ingredients

- 4 pita breads
- 200 g turkey meat
- salt
- pepper
- 50 g rocket
- 10 cocktail tomatoes
- 1/2 onion
- 1 clove of garlic
- 200 g yogurt

Preparation

1. Warm up the pita breads in the hot air fryer.
2. Cut the turkey meat into bite-sized pieces and grill on the hot air fryer's grill plate for about 10-15 minutes.
3. Wash the rocket and quarter the tomatoes, cut the onion into thin rings.
4. Sauté the onion rings in the hot air fryer for 3 minutes .
5. Mix the yogurt with a pressed clove of garlic, salt and pepper.
6. Fill the warmed pita breads with the turkey meat, vegetables and yogurt sauce.

Chicken curry skewers from the hot air fryer

- Cooking time More than 60 min
- Servings: 4

Ingredients

- 4 chicken breasts
- for the marinade:
- 100 ml coconut milk
- 3 tbsp curry powder
- 1 bunch of coriander
- 10 tbsp yogurt
- salt
- pepper

Preparation

1. Clean the chicken and cut lengthways into strips. Wash the coriander, dry it well and chop it finely.

2. Mix all ingredients for the marinade well. Put the chicken strips in and leave to marinate for several hours.
3. Place the strips of meat on the Airfryer skewers.
4. Grill in the hot air fryer at 180 ° C for about 10 minutes.

Fried chicken salad from the hot air fryer

- Cooking time 15 to 30 min
- Servings: 4

Ingredients

- 2 chicken breasts (approx. 200 g each)
- salt
- Pepper (from the mill)
- Lemon juice
- Parsley (chopped)
- Oil (for frying)
- Leaf lettuce (of your choice)
- 8 cherry tomatoes

For the panier:

- Flour (smooth)
- Breadcrumbs
- 1 egg

For the marinade:

- 2 tbsp vinegar
- 4 tbsp vegetable oil
- salt

- Pepper (from the mill)
- Icing sugar
- mustard

Preparation

1. For the fried chicken salad from the hot air fryer, first finely chop the parsley. Cut the meat into strips about 3 cm long or cubes. Rub with parsley, salt, pepper and a little lemon juice.
2. Set up a breading line: first a plate with flour, then one with a beaten egg and finally one with breadcrumbs. Bread the chicken pieces with flour, egg and breadcrumbs.
3. Bake with a little oil at 150 °C for about 7 minutes in the hot air fryer.
4. In the meantime, prepare the salad. Mix all ingredients well for the marinade. Wash the lettuce and spin dry. Mix with the cherry tomatoes and marinate everything. Distribute on plates and place the fried chicken pieces on top. Serve the fried chicken salad from the air fryer immediately.

Chicken breast on grilled vegetables from the air fryer

- Cooking time 30 to 60 min
- Servings: 2

Ingredients

- 2 chicken breasts
- 1 sprig (s) of rosemary
- 2-3 sprig (s) of thyme
- 1 1/2 peppers
- 1/2 zucchini
- 1/2 clove of garlic
- 1 onion
- 4 cherry tomatoes
- 1-2 tbsp vegetable oil
- salt
- Pepper (from the mill)

For the pesto:
- 2 handfuls of basil
- 1 handful of parsley
- 50 g pine nuts

- 30 g parmesan cheese
- 125 ml of olive oil
- some salt

Preparation

1. For the chicken breast on grilled vegetables, first clean the chicken (do not cut off the skin), salt and pepper.
2. Heat vegetable oil and fry the chicken breasts from the skin side for about 2 minutes, then turn them over, add the rosemary and fry for another 2 minutes.
3. Place the meat on the grill plate or in the baking pan and place in the hot air fryer at 120 ° C for about 20-25 minutes .
4. Toast the pine nuts in a pan without oil until they are fragrant. Mix with the plucked parsley, the plucked basil, grated Parmesan, a little salt and 25 ml of olive oil to make a pesto. Gradually pour in the remaining olive oil.
5. Peel the onion and cut into wedges. Wash the zucchini, cut off the stalk and cut in half lengthways. Remove cores. Halve on both sides and cut into thin sticks. Core the paprika, cut away the stalk and cut the

pulp into thin strips. Halve the tomatoes. Peel the garlic and cut into thin slices. Peel off the thyme and chop finely.
6. Fry the onion in hot olive oil. Add paprika and fry for about 1 1/2 minutes. Then add the zucchini and garlic. After another 1 1/2 minutes add the tomatoes and season the vegetables with thyme, salt and pepper. Remove from heat and let stand for about 10 minutes.
7. The chicken breast on grilled vegetables with pesto cause.

Air Fryer BBQ Wings

- Preparation time 30mins
- Cooking time 60mins
- Servings 4

Ingredients

- 2 pounds of chicken wings
- 1 tablespoon brown sugar
- 1 teaspoon of sea salt
- 1 teaspoon garlic powder
- 1 teaspoon smoked paprika
- 1/2 teaspoon ground black pepper
- 1/4 teaspoon baking powder
- olive oil spray
- Barbecue sauce

Preparation

1. Mix spices and baking powder in a small bowl
2. Dry the wings with a paper towel.
3. Rub the mixture on the wings until well covered and place the wings on the flyer rack.
4. Spritz olive oil and wing spray
5. Preheat the fryer to 390 degrees, add wings to the fryer, cook for 25-30 minutes, and turn the pan half-turn during cooking. According to the thermometer, the internal temperature should be at least 165 degrees.
6. Remove from the flyer and polish with your favorite barbecue sauce!

Ham-wrapped turkey

- preparation time 15mins
- cooking time 30mins
- servings 2

Ingredients

- 300 g turkey fillet
- Honey mustard
- Mountain air ham
- Oil

Preparation

1. For the turkey wrapped in ham, coat the turkey fillets with honey mustard.
2. Wrap with mountain air ham. Fry slowly on both sides in a little oil over low heat.
3. Serve the turkey wrapped in ham with a side dish.

Jamaican jerk turkey

- preparation time 30mins
- cooking time 60mins
- servings 6

Ingredients

- 750 g turkey breast (schnitzel)
- For the jerk marinade:
- 1/2 cup (s) of orange juice
- 1/2 cup (s) of vinegar
- 1/2 cup (s) soy sauce
- 1/4 cup (s) of olive oil
- jalapeno (diced)
- 1 tbsp sugar
- 1 teaspoon salt
- 1 teaspoon thyme
- 1 teaspoon cinnamon
- 1/2 teaspoon nutmeg
- tbsp new spice
- 1 tbsp ginger (fresh)

- 3 cloves of garlic (crushed)
- 4 spring onions (cut into thin strips)

Preparation

1. First, make the marinade for the Jamaican Jerk Turkey. To do this, mix all the marinade ingredients in a flat glass bowl. Put 1/2 cup aside and use later as a dip and for glazing.
2. Put in the schnitzel and chill for at least 30 minutes - preferably overnight.
3. Grill the Jamaican Jerk Turkey for 15-20 minutes until the meat is no longer pink.

Turkey in the port wine bath

- preparation time 15mins
- cooking time 30mins

Ingredients

- 500 g turkey breast
- 2 peppers (yellow)
- 1/4 l port wine
- 2 tbsp mascarpone

Preparation

1. Chop the turkey breast, season with salt and pepper, cut the bell pepper into large strips.

Tuna with a fruity cucumber salad

- preparation time 20mins
- servings 2

Ingredients

- 2 tuna fillets approx. 130 g each
- salt
- pepper from the mill
- 2 tsp olive oil
- 200 g cucumber
- 150 g Chinese cabbage
- 4 tbsp lime juice
- 4 tbsp chilli chicken sauce
- 4 tbsp orange juice
- 4 tbsp spring onion rings

Preparation

1. Salt and pepper the tuna fillets. Olive oil in a coated
2. Heat a pan, fry the fish fillets in it for approx. 2 - 3 minutes on each side. Wash the cucumber with the skin and cut into thin slices or slice.
3. Wash and clean the Chinese cabbage and cut into thin strips.
4. Mix the cucumber, Chinese cabbage, lime juice, chilli chicken sauce, orange juice and spring onion rings and season with salt. Arrange the tuna fillets on the salad and serve.

BEEF RECIPES

Meat skewers with letscho from the air fryer

- Cooking time 15 to 30 min
- Servings: 4

Ingredients

- 500 g pork (e.g. neck)
- 1 shallot

For the marinade:
- 2 cloves of garlic
- 3 tbsp paprika powder
- 2 tbsp ketchup
- 4 tbsp vegetable oil

For the letscho:
- 6 peppers
- 1 onion
- 500 g tomatoes (peeled, canned)
- 125 ml of water
- 1 pinch of paprika powder

- salt
- pepper

Preparation

1. For the meat skewers with Letscho from the hot air fryer, first clean the pork and cut into large cubes. Peel the garlic and finely chop or press. Wash the peppers, remove the seeds and the stalk and cut the pulp into large cubes. Peel the onion and shallot. Roughly chop the onion. Cut the shallot into wide wedges.
2. Mix all ingredients for the marinade. Mix the meat cubes with it and marinate in it for at least half an hour.
3. Heat oil in a pan. Sweat the onions in it. Add 2/3 of the peppers. Season with salt, pepper and paprika. Deglaze with the water and add the tomatoes and juice.
4. Drain on the meat cubes and place on the skewers with the remaining paprika and shallots.
5. Grill in the hot air fryer at 180 ° C for 5-10 minutes. Serve meat skewers with Letscho from the air fryer.

Frittata with corn, paprika and grilled turkey cubes

- Cooking time 15 to 30 min
- Servings: 4

Ingredients

- 5 eggs
- 1/2 can (s) of corn
- 1 pepper
- 150 g turkey fillet (diced)
- 1 clove (s) of garlic (finely chopped)
- 2 tbsp parmesan
- 2 handfuls of herbs (chives and parsley)
- salt
- pepper
- 1 spring onion

Preparation

1. For the frittata with corn, paprika and grilled turkey cubes from the hot air fryer, cut the turkey meat into small cubes and grill with a little oil in the hot air fryer for about 5 minutes.
2. Put the finely chopped garlic, corn, finely chopped spring onions, chopped peppers in an ovenproof dish, and let simmer for about 5 minutes in the hot air fryer. Mix the meat with the vegetables.
3. Whisk eggs and parmesan in a bowl. Season with salt and pepper and pour over the meat-vegetable mixture.
4. Bake the frittata with corn, paprika and grilled turkey cubes for about 20 minutes at 180 ° C in the hot air fryer. The frittata with sweet corn, peppers and grilled turkey cubes from the air fryer before serving, sprinkle chopped basil.

Express beef roulades in a caper cream sauce

Ingredients

- 4 slices of Beiried (approx. 180 g each)
- 100 g bacon (without rind)
- 4 pickles
- 100 g leeks
- 300 g cream cheese
- 100 ml beef soup
- 1 tbsp caper berries (without stalk)
- 1 tbsp tarragon mustard (or Dijon mustard)
- salt
- Pepper (from the mill)
- olive oil
- 250 g pasta (of your choice

Preparation

1. Put on a saucepan with pasta water. The Airfryer to 165 ° C preheat.
2. Pound the Beiried thinly, season with salt, pepper and brush with a little mustard. Cut the bacon, cucumber and leek into thin strips and divide between the beetroot slices.
3. Fold the meat on the sides and roll it into roulades. Secure with skewers or toothpicks and cook in the hot air fryer's baking pan with a dash of olive oil at 165 ° C for about 15 minutes.
4. Beat the cream cheese with the soup and the capers until smooth and add to the roulades. Cook for another 10 minutes.
5. Simultaneously, cook the pasta until al dente according to the instructions on the package, strain and mix with a little butter if necessary.
6. Arrange with the pasta on plates and serve.

Beef roulades from the air fryer

- Cooking time 30 to 60 min
- Servings: 4

Ingredients

- 800g Rinderrouladen
- 4 Sour cucumbers
- 4 slices of ham
- 4 tsp mustard
- Salt pepper
- 4 wooden sticks
- 4 small carrots
- 4 small potatoes
- 2 parsnips
- 1 Red onion
- 1 tbsp oil
- 1 teaspoon fresh rosemary

Preparation

1. Cut carrots, parsnips, potatoes, and onions. Add oil, salt, pepper, and rosemary, mix and cook at 180 ° C for 10 minutes in the s Air fryer.
2. Now spread the beef roulades. Season with salt and pepper and brush with a teaspoon of mustard put a slice of ham on the roulade and an acid cucumber on top. Roll up and fix it with a wooden skewer. Kitchen yarn also works great for fixing.
3. Place the roulades on the pre-cooked vegetables and place them in the hot air fryer at 180 ° C for 15 minutes. Finished!

Beef steak with onion vegetables

- Total time 25 min
- servings 4

Ingredients

- 4 onions
- 1 tbsp butter
- 2 tbsp vegetable oil
- salt
- pepper from the mill
- 4 steaks of approx. 200

Preparation

1. Peel the onions, cut in half and cut into strips. Fry in hot butter and 1 tablespoon of oil over mild heat for 8-10 minutes until golden brown. Salt, pepper and remove from the pan.
2. Flatten the steaks slightly, season with salt, pepper and fry in the pan in the remaining

hot oil for 2-4 minutes on each side (depending on your preference). Finally, add the onions again, let them get hot and serve.

Corned beef sandwich

- Preparation: 30 min
- servings 4

Ingredients

- 500 g corned beef
- 3 gherkins
- 200 g watercress
- 300 g cooked beetroot
- 4 tbsp mayonnaise
- 1 tsp medium-hot mustard
- 8 slices whole-grain rye bread
- cayenne pepper
- 4 slices sliced cheese

Preparation

1. Cut the corned beef into 0.7 cm thick slices. Drain the pickles well and cut lengthways into thin slices. Wash the cress, sort, clean and spin dry. Peel and coarsely grate the beetroot. Mix the mayonnaise with the mustard. Preheat the oven to grill function. Toast the bread slices and brush half of the slices with mayonnaise and season with cayenne pepper.
2. Spread the beetroot and the pickled gurgles on top, cover each with 1-2 slices of corned beef and 1 slice of cheese and let it melt briefly under the hot oven grill. Take out, spread the cress on top, cover with a second slice of bread and serve fixed with a wooden skewer.

Grilled beef steak

Ingredients

- 4 slices of Beiried (beef)
- 6 tbsp oil
- 1 sprig (s) of rosemary (fresh)
- salt
- pepper
- Herb butter

Preparation

1. Mix a marinade for the grilled beef steak from oil, salt, pepper and the fresh rosemary needles. Brush the steaks on both sides. Place on the hot grid and roast for only a few minutes on both sides so that the meat is still pink on the inside.
2. You can also cook the steak in a very hot pan.

3. Serve a homemade herb butter with the grilled beef steak.
4. Straw apples and peas with ham go well with the grilled beef steak.

Sliced beef

Ingredients

- 500 g beef fillet
- 2 tbsp frying fat
- 1 pc onion
- 1 clove (s) of garlic
- 1 tbsp butter
- 1 tbsp flour
- 1/4 l soup
- 1/4 l beer
- salt
- pepper
- thyme

Preparation

1. Cut the beef fillet into strips, heat the frying fat and quickly fry the meat. Take out of the pan and keep warm; Finely chop the onion and garlic and translate

them in butter. Dust with flour and lightly brown. Deglaze with soup and beer and season with salt, pepper and thyme. Add the meat and cook for 20 minutes.

Wok vegetables with meat

Ingredients

- 400 g pork
- 580 g wok vegetables (igloo)
- 6 tbsp rapeseed oil
- marjoram
- thyme
- salt
- pepper

Preparation

1. First, for the wok vegetables with meat, dice the pork and soak in a mixture of rapeseed oil, salt, pepper, marjoram, and thyme. Let it steep for at least 3 hours, preferably overnight.
2. Put the pork in a wok without adding any more oil and sear it. Add the wok

vegetables and wait for the water to evaporate.
3. Then sear everything together again. The wok vegetables with meat taste even with salt and pepper and serve.

Beef and green beans salad

- preparation time 15 to 30 min
- servings 4

Ingredients

- 300 g beef (lean, ready-cooked)
- 1 kg of fisoles
- 2 spring onions (very fresh)
- 20 g horseradish
- 1 pc. Paprika (red)
- vinegar
- Pumpkin seed oil
- salt
- pepper

Preparation

1. For the beef and green beans salad, wash the green beans carefully. Then cut or break into small pieces. Put water in a saucepan and bring to the boil, season with salt and insert the beans' pieces. Let simmer in salted water for a while. Then remove it with a scoop and let it cool.
2. In the meantime, wash the onion, dry it and cut it into fine strips. Also, use green.
3. Peel the horseradish and tear finely.
4. Wash the peppers and cut into fine strips.
5. Cut the meat into fine, bite-sized picces.
6. Mix the green beans, meat, bell pepper and onion. Marinate with vinegar and oil, mix in the horseradish and season with salt and pepper to taste.
7. Fresh bread is an excellent accompaniment to the beef and green bean salad.

Meatballs with green salad

- Preparation: 30 min
- servings 4

Ingredients

- 1 stale bun
- 125 g mozzarella (9% fat)
- 3 stems parsley
- 1 clove of garlic
- 500 g beefsteak hack
- 1 egg
- 1 tsp hot mustard
- salt
- pepper
- 1 tbsp rapeseed oil
- 150 g mixed leaf salad
- 200 g blue seedless grapes
- 2 tbsp orange juice
- 1 tsp liquid honey
- Dijon mustard

- 3 tbsp olive oil

Preparation

1. Soak the rolls. Drain the mozzarella and cut into small cubes. Wash parsley, shake dry, pluck leaves.
2. Peel and press the garlic. Squeeze out the bun. Knead with garlic, mince, egg, hot mustard, salt and pepper. Shape the mixture into balls, flatten them, place 1 piece of mozzarella on top, cover with the meat dough. Shape the balls again, pressing 1 parsley leaf on each of them.
3. Heat the rapeseed oil in a pan and fry the balls around medium heat until golden brown. Reduce heat and finish cooking.
4. In the meantime, wash and spin the salad. Wash grapes and cut in half. For the dressing stir together orange juice, honey, Dijon mustard and olive oil, season with salt and pepper. Mix the salad with the grapes, arrange plates with meatballs, and drizzle with dressing.

Hearty turnip and carrot stew with beef

- Preparation: 30 min
- Total time 2 h

Ingredients

- 4 onions
- 1 clove of garlic
- 1 piece celeriac (200 g)
- 2 tbsp butter (30 g)
- 800 g beef goulash
- 1 l hot vegetable broth
- 1 bay leaf
- 2 cloves
- 1 tsp dried marjoram
- salt
- pepper
- 1 turnip (700 g)
- 3 carrots
- ½ fret parsley (10 g)
- 1-piece fresh horseradish for garnish

Preparation

1. Peel and chop the onion and garlic. Clean, peel, wash and finely dice the celery. Heat the butter in a saucepan. Fry the onion and celery in it for about 5 minutes over high heat. Stir and scrape the roasted ingredients from the bottom. Take the onion and celery out of the pot.
2. Put the meat in the saucepan and fry for 5 minutes over high heat. Add the garlic and fry for 1–2 minutes. Then deglaze with 50 ml of stock and simmer for 3–4 minutes, stirring occasionally.
3. Return the onion and celery to the pot. Add bay leaf, cloves, marjoram and season with salt and pepper. Cover and simmer over low heat for about 70 minutes, stirring occasionally.
4. In the meantime, wash and peel the turnip and cut into cubes approx. 2 x 2 cm. Peel, wash and chop the carrots. Wash the parsley, shake dry and roughly chop the leaves.
5. Then add the turnip and carrots and simmer covered for another 15 minutes.

Remove the bay leaf and cloves. Remove the beef and ⅔ of the turnip and the carrots with a slotted spoon. Mix the rest of the soup with a hand blender. Add the meat and vegetables again and bring everything to a boil.
6. Finally, peel the horseradish and grate finely. Season the turnip stew with salt and pepper. Serve the turnip stew and garnish with horseradish and parsley.

Smart beef goulash basic recipe

- Preparation: 2 h
- serving 4

ingredients

- 250 g carrots (3 carrots)
- 150 g celeriac (1 piece)
- 3 onions
- 2 tbsp rapeseed oil
- 600 g beef goulash
- 45 g tomato paste (3 tbsp)
- 600 ml of meat soup
- ½ tsp peppercorns
- salt
- pepper
- 2 tsp paprika powder
- 1 tsp marjoram
- 1 branch rosemary

Preparation

1. Clean, peel and wash the carrots and celery and cut into cubes. Peel the onions and cut into strips.
2. Heat oil in a pot. Fry the meat in it for 5 minutes over high heat. Add the vegetables and fry vigorously for 5 minutes, stirring and scraping the roasted substances from the bottom. Add tomato paste and let caramelize for 4 minutes while stirring; the tomato paste is lightly browned and gives the goulash a nice brown colour. Then deglaze with 50 ml of stock and simmer for 3–4 minutes, stirring occasionally.
3. Pour in the rest of the broth, season with salt, pepper, peppercorns, paprika powder, marjoram and rosemary. Cover and simmer over low heat for about 1 1/2 hours until the sauce is creamy, stirring occasionally. Season the goulash with salt and pepper.

Meat vegetable strudel

- Cooking time: 60 min
- servings 4

Ingredients

For the fullness:
- 150 g mixed vegetables (3x)
- 200 g minced meat (mixed)
- 60 g dumpling bread
- 1 tbsp sunflower oil
- 30 g onion
- 1 pc egg
- 1 piece of egg white
- 1 tbsp parsley
- salt
- Pepper, marjoram

For painting:
- 1 pc yolk

Dough shell:
- 330 g puff pastry (1 package)

Preparation

1. For the meat and vegetable strudel, cook the vegetables briefly. Finely chop and roast the onion.
2. For the meat filling, soften the dumpling bread with a little water and finely chop the parsley.
3. Mix all the ingredients for the meat mixture well, then add the vegetables.
4. Place the puff pastry on a floured strudel or tea towel, shape the filling into a roll, place on the dough and roll-up.
5. Place on a baking tray covered with baking paper and coat with the yolk.
6. Bake in the oven at 200 ° C for about 40 minutes.
7. Then cut open the meat and vegetable strudel and serve.

Roast steak perfectly

- Cooking time 15 to 30 min

Ingredients

- 600 g beiried (or 3 steaks a 200 g)
- 2 tbsp oil
- Seasoning mix or marinade

Preparation

1. For the steaks, preheat the oven to 110 ° C (no convection).
2. Heat the oil in a pan, fry the seasoned or marinated steaks in the hot oil for about 3-4 minutes, remove and place on a plate.
3. Let it steep in the oven for about 10 minutes.

PORK RECIPES

Roast pork from the air fryer

- Cooking time More than 60 min
- Servings: 4

Ingredients

- 1200 g pork tuft (alternatively square)
- 3 cloves of garlic
- Salt (coarse)
- 1 teaspoon peppercorns (black)
- 2 cloves
- 1 1/2 tbsp vegetable oil
- 1 teaspoon rosemary
- 5 pumpkin seeds
- 1 bunch of soup vegetables
- 1 bay leaf
- 200 ml of beer
- 200 g leeks
- 200 ml beef soup

Preparation

1. For the roast pork from the air fryer, first strip off the rosemary. Peel the garlic. Grind both together with pumpkin seeds, cloves, salt and pepper. Stir in the vegetable oil.
2. Cut the pig's head into a check pattern on the rind. Massage in the spice paste. Place the rind down in the baking pan of the hot air fryer. Add about 1 cm high boiling water. Fry at 200 ° C for about 15 minutes. Turn the roast pork over and cook for another 15 minutes.
3. In the meantime, peel the soup vegetables and cut into thin slices. Add to roast pork. Add the bay leaf as well. Empty the beer over the roast pork. Slide into the hot air fryer for 45 minutes. In between, pour the gravy over and over again.
4. Meanwhile, wash the leek and cut into large pieces. Add to the roast pork with the beef soup. Fry again at 175 ° C for 45 minutes and pour over the gravy several times.

5. Remove the meat and leek. Puree the sauce finely and thicken if necessary. Serve roast pork from the air fryer.

Spare ribs from the air fryer

- Cooking time More than 60 min
- Servings: 2

Ingredients

- 2 spare ribs

For the marinade:
- 3 tbsp olive oil
- 2 tbsp honey
- 4 tbsp soy sauce
- 1 1/2 tbsp sugar (brown)
- 1/2 can (s) tomatoes (in small pieces)
- 1 teaspoon chili powder
- 5 tbsp apple juice

Preparation

1. For the spare ribs from the hot air fryer, first remove the silver skin on the bone of the spare ribs. To do this, slightly incise the skin and pull it off with a strong pull.

2. Mix all ingredients for the marinade well. Massage the ribs with it and let it marinate overnight.
3. Drain the marinade and the spareribs at 150 ° C for about 60-90 minutes in the Airfryer grill.

Pork rack fried in water

- Preparation time 5mins
- Cooking time 15mins
- Servings 4

Ingredients

- 6 pork chops
- dose of aged cachaça
- 1 tablespoon of turmeric
- 1 teaspoon salt
- 1 cup of water
- Pepper to taste

Preparation

1. With the aid of a knife, make light and diagonal cuts in the slices, without piercing them;
2. In a container, season the chops with pepper, salt and saffron, spreading well on both sides;

3. Add the cachaça and leave the container in the refrigerator for about 30 minutes;
4. In a heated skillet, place the chops and let them fry for 3 minutes on each side;
5. Add half the cup of water, then turn the chops and add the rest of the water;
6. Cover the pan, let it cook for 1 minute and then turn the steaks;
7. Transfer to a plate and serve.

Fried pork rack

Ingredients

- 4 pork chops
- 4 chopped garlic cloves
- 1 teaspoon of oregano
- 1 teaspoon cumin
- 1 teaspoon of dye
- 1 teaspoon salt
- 300 ml of oil
- 1 lemon juice

Preparation

1. Spread the garlic, oregano, cumin, dye and salt in the chops and let it rest for a few minutes;
2. In a saucepan, heat the oil and then place the pieces of steak for frying;
3. When browned on both sides, remove the oil and serve.

Stuffed meat roll

- Cooking time 60 min

Ingredients

- 1 kg of meat (beef or pork)
- 2 rolls
- 3 pcs. Onions
- 3 toe (s) of garlic
- 1 tbsp mustard
- salt
- pepper
- 1 package of sauerkraut

Preparation

1. For the meat roll, mince the meat and mix with finely chopped onions, garlic, mustard, salt, pepper and a little parsley.
2. In the meantime, let the rolls soak a little, press them out and mix in as well.
3. Spread the mixture about 2 cm thick on a baking sheet and cover with sauerkraut.

Roll up the foil and bake on a greased baking sheet in an oven preheated to 175 °C for about 45 minutes.
4. Shortly before the end of the baking time, open the foil a little so that the meat roll can take on a little colour.
5. Cut the finished meat roll into thick slices and enjoy while still hot!

Pork stew

- Cooking time 60 min

Ingredients

- 500 g pork (lean)
- 1 pc. Paprika (red)
- 1 pc. Paprika (green)
- 1 onion (large)
- 200 g mushrooms
- Butter (for frying)
- 1/4 l sour cream
- salt
- pepper
- 1 teaspoon paprika powder
- garlic
- 1 teaspoon flour

Preparation

1. For the pork goulash, cut the meat into pieces approx. 1 cm wide and 3 cm long.

1. Finely chop the onions, cut the peppers into strips and the mushrooms into flakes.
2. Briefly toast the salted and peppered meat in hot butter, remove and place on a plate.
3. Let the onions lightly roast in the frying residue, add the peppers and mushrooms, and let them simmer until soft.
4. Dust with flour and add garlic, salt, pepper, paprika powder and sour cream. Bring the whole thing to the boil, as the sauce should have thickened a little before adding the meat again to heat it.
5. Then serve the pork goulash hot.

Caribbean style spare ribs

- preparation time 5mins
- cooking time 15mins

ingredients

- 2 spare ribs
- 50 ml peanut oil
- 100 ml coconut milk
- 3 tbsp pineapple juice
- 1/2 teaspoon ginger
- 1/2 tbsp curry paste (green)
- 1/2 stick (s) lemongrass
- salt
- pepper
- Honey (for glazing)
- 1 handful of basil

Preparation

1. For the Caribbean spare ribs, rinse the meat and pat dry.
2. Mix a marinade of peanut oil, coconut milk, lemongrass, pineapple juice, green curry paste, basil and ginger.
3. Put the spare ribs in the marinade and let them steep for a few hours, preferably overnight.
4. Then remove too much marinade from the spare ribs. Salt and pepper.
5. The Spareribs Caribbean style put on the grill and cook about 5-7 minutes. Always turn around.

Spare ribs the hell of a way

Ingredients

- 2 spare ribs
- 50 ml chilli oil
- 50 ml soy sauce
- 1 tbsp lemon juice
- 2 teaspoons of cayenne pepper
- 2 tbsp Tabasco
- salt
- pepper
- Honey (for glazing)

Preparation

1. For the spicy spare ribs, rinse the meat and pat dry.
2. Mix a marinade of chili oil, cayenne pepper, Tabasco, soy sauce and lemon juice.

3. Place the spare ribs in the marinade and let them steep for a few hours, preferably overnight.
4. Then remove too much marinade from the spare ribs. Salt and pepper.
5. The Sparribs on the grill and grill place about 5-7 minutes. Always turn around.

Pork in cider batter

- preparation time 15mins
- cooking time 30mins

ingredients

- 1 pork fillet
- mustard
- Horseradish (grated)
- salt
- pepper
- Fat (for frying)
- 250 g of flour
- 3 eggs
- 1 pinch of salt
- 1 pinch of cinnamon
- Must (depending on consistency)

Preparation

1. For the pork in cider dough, first mix the dough ingredients and let rest for 45-60 minutes.
2. Slice the meat and rub mustard, horseradish, salt and pepper. Pull through the dough and bake in the hot fat. The pork in Mostteig Drain before serving on paper towels.

Pork medallions

- preparation time 15mins
- cooking time 30mins
- servings 4

Ingredients

- 1 kg of pork sirloin
- Caraway seed
- salt
- pepper
- 1 clove of garlic (pressed)
- oil
- 1/16 l beer
- 1/4 l gravy

Preparation

1. For the pork medallions, cut the pork lung roast into pieces and season with caraway seeds, salt, pepper and garlic, fry in oil and set aside. Deglaze the roast

residue with beer and gravy and briefly bring to the boil. Pour the sauce over the meat.

Baked Hawaiian schnitzel

Ingredients

- 4 pork schnitzel (from the upper shell, approx. 200 g each)
- salt
- pepper from the mill
- 2 tbsp olive oil
- 8 slices pineapple (can)
- 4 slices gouda cheese
- pink pepper
- frize salad sheet for the garnish

Preparation

1. Wash the schnitzel, pat dry, halve each, season with salt and pepper. Heat the oil in a pan and fry the meat for 1–2 minutes on each side.
2. Place the schnitzel on a baking rack and put one slice of pineapple on each. Cover

with the cheese and bake in the preheated oven at 220 ° C top heat for about 5 minutes.
3. Sprinkle the Hawaiian schnitzel with pink pepper and garnish with frisée.

Pork steaks with chanterelles

- Preparation time 15mins
- Cooking time 30mins
- Servings 4

Ingredients

- 4 pork steaks
- 8 spring onions
- 2 tbsp olive oil
- 15 days chanterelles (optionally also mushrooms)
- salt
- pepper
- 4 potatoes

Preparation

1. For the pork steaks with chanterelles, salt and pepper the pork steaks. Fry both sides in oil in a non-stick pan. Remove steaks and keep warm.

2. Fry the spring onions slowly in the pan. Add the chanterelles and season with salt and pepper. Cook the potatoes with the skin on. Cut in the middle and fry on both sides in a pan with a little oil.

Fried pork rack

Ingredients

- 4 pork chops
- 4 chopped garlic cloves
- 1 teaspoon of oregano
- 1 teaspoon cumin
- 1 teaspoon of dye
- 1 teaspoon salt
- 300 ml of oil
- 1 lemon juice

Preparation

4. Spread the garlic, oregano, cumin, dye and salt in the chops and let it rest for a few minutes;
5. In a saucepan, heat the oil and then place the pieces of steak for frying;
6. When browned on both sides, remove the oil and serve.

Boneless drumstick in a simple oven

- preparation time 15mins
- cooking time 30mins
- servings 2

Ingredients

- 1 onion
- Olive oil to taste
- 1 kg of boneless drumstick
- Salt to taste
- 150 g bacon

Preparation

1. On a platter, place the onion cut into medium slices and drizzle with olive oil;
2. Remove the skin from the drumstick, season with salt and wrap with the bacon strips;

3. Transfer to the platter and bake in a preheated oven at 180 ° C for half an hour.

VEGETABLE RECIPES

Mini peppers with goat cheese from the hot air fryer

- Cooking time 15 to 30 min
- Servings: 8

Ingredients

- 8 mini peppers (or snack peppers)
- 1/2 tbsp olive oil
- 1/2 tbsp Italian herbs (dried)
- 1 teaspoon pepper (black, freshly ground)
- **100 g goat cheese (soft, cut into 8 pieces)**

Preparation

1. For the mini peppers with goat cheese, cut off the mini peppers' top and remove the seeds and the white skin.

2. Mix the olive oil with the Italian herbs and pepper in a deep plate. Turn the goat cheese pieces in the oil.
3. Put a piece of goat cheese in each mini pepper and place the mini peppers side by side in the basket. Slide the basket into the Philips Airfryer air fryer and set the timer to 8-10 minutes. Bake the mini peppers at 200 ° C until the cheese has melted.
4. The mini-peppers with goat cheese on small plates as appetizers or snacks served.

Potato and vegetable chips from the hot air fryer

- Cooking time 30 to 60 min

Ingredients

- 100 g potatoes
- tbsp rapeseed oil
- salt
- pepper
- paprika

preparation

1. For the potato and vegetable chips, peel the potatoes and cut into fine slices with the food processor.
2. Leave the potato slices in cold water for 20 minutes so that the starch can come out.
3. Then pat the slices dry with a cloth and mix with the oil.
4. The Airfryer to 160 ° C provide.

5. Put the potatoes in the Quick Clean Basket, close and bake for about 20 minutes until crispy brown.
6. When you take the potato and vegetable chips out of the hot air fryer, season to taste.

Potato gratin with wild garlic

- Cooking time More than 60 min
- Servings: 4

Ingredients

- 330 g potatoes (waxy)
- 1 handful of wild garlic
- 1 1/2 peppers
- 1/2 stick (s) leek
- 1 1/2 spring onions
- 2 eggs (large)
- 165 g sour cream
- 130 ml whipped cream
- 1/2 teaspoon mustard
- 1 pinch of nutmeg (freshly grated)
- salt
- Pepper (freshly ground)
- Butter (for the mould)
- Cheese (grated, for sprinkling)

Preparation

1. For the potato gratin with wild garlic from the hot air fryer, wash the wild garlic, dry it well and chop it finely. Peel the potatoes and cut them into thin slices. Wash the peppers, remove the stalk and white skin and cut the pulp into cubes. Wash the spring onions and cut them into thin rings.
2. Whisk the eggs with sour cream, whipped cream, mustard, nutmeg, salt and pepper.
3. Grease the baking pan of the hot air fryer. Fill in the vegetables and potato slices in layers. Pour the egg mixture over it. Finally, sprinkle the grated cheese on top.
4. Bake for about 60 minutes at 180 ° C in the hot air fryer. Portion potato gratin with wild garlic from the air fryer and serve.

Asparagus lasagna from the hot air fryer

- Cooking time 30 to 60 min
- Servings: 4

Ingredients

- 9 sheets of lasagne
- 500 g asparagus (green)
- 500 g asparagus (white)
- 2 tbsp butter
- 500 ml of milk
- 2 tbsp flour
- salt
- Pepper (from the mill)
- Nutmeg (freshly grated)
- oregano
- 100 g parmesan cheese

Preparation

1. For the asparagus lasagne from the hot air fryer, first peel the white asparagus and cut off 2-3 cm at the bottom. The green asparagus does not have to be peeled, just cut off 2-3 cm at the bottom.
2. Cook the asparagus in salted water with a little butter until al dente.
3. For the béchamel sauce, melt the butter in a saucepan, stir in the flour and mix with the milk to form a creamy sauce. Season to taste with salt, pepper, nutmeg and oregano.
4. Grease the hot air fryer's baking pan and pour in layer by layer of lasagne sheets, asparagus and bechamel sauce until all the ingredients are used up. The last layer should be bechamel sauce. Scatter the parmesan on top.

Pumpkin fritters from the air fryer

Ingredients

- 1 pc. Pumpkin (Hokkaido, nutmeg or Langer from Naples)
- 1 egg
- 100 g cream cheese
- 70 g breadcrumbs
- 1 bunch of parsley (small, chopped)
- salt
- Pepper (from the mill)
- Nutmeg (ground)
- olive oil

Preparation

1. Halve and core the pumpkin. Grate coarsely, season with salt and let steep for about 10 minutes.
2. Squeeze the pumpkin well and mix in a bowl with the cream cheese, egg,

breadcrumbs, chopped parsley and the spices. Let it soak for another 5 minutes.
3. Shape balls with wet hands, flatten them and fry them in the hot air fryer (with a teaspoon of olive oil) at 180 °C for 6-7 minutes on the grill plate. Turn and fry for another 6-7 minutes on the second side.
4. Keep the finished pumpkin pancakes warm and repeat with the remaining mixture until everything is used up and made into pumpkin pancakes.

Spinach strudel from the hot air fryer

- Cooking time 15 to 30 min
- Servings: 4

Ingredients

- 1. packet of puff pastry
- 170 g sour cream
- 750 g spinach leaves
- 250 g sheep cheese (crumbled)
- 2 tbsp butter (melted)
- 4 cloves of garlic (peeled, mashed)
- salt
- pepper

Preparation

1. Pick the spinach leaves properly and wash them well in cold water.
2. Bring salted water to a boil in a large saucepan, add the spinach and blanch (scald) for about 1 minute. Drain and soak

in ice water immediately, otherwise, it will lose its beautiful green colour.
3. Then cut into fine strips and mix with the crumbled sheep's cheese, crushed garlic and spices.
4. Roll out the puff pastry and spread the sour cream in the middle. Spread the spinach mixture in the middle of the dough, fold in the sides, roll up, seal the ends well.
5. Place the spinach strudel on the grill cup and brush with the melted butter.
6. Bake in the hot air fryer at 180 ° C for about 25 minutes.

Baked vegetables from the air fryer

Ingredients

- 1 broccoli
- 1 zucchini
- 250 g mushrooms

For breading:

- 150 g flour (smooth)
- 200 g of breadcrumbs
- 2 eggs (large)
- Salt
- 1 teaspoon sunflower oil

Preparation

1. Cut up the broccoli with a small knife, remove the stalk and cut the broccoli roses in half if necessary.
2. Boil over in some boiling salted water for about 20 seconds, then cool in ice-cold water (= blanching). Let dry on kitchen paper.

3. Cut off the ends of the zucchini, cut the rest diagonally into approx. 1 cm thick slices. Clean the mushrooms, halve or quarter the large mushrooms.
4. First turn the vegetables in flour, pull them through the beaten, salted eggs and finally bread them with the breadcrumbs.
5. Put the vegetables in the hot air fryer, add a little oil to the cooking space and bake at 185 ° C for about 8-10 minutes until crispy.
6. Arrange and serve with a dip of your choice.

Cooked oven vegetables from the air fryer

- Cooking time 15 to 30 min
- Servings: 2

Ingredients

- 1 bell pepper (red)
- 1 bell pepper (yellow)
- 1 zucchini
- 1 onion (red)
- Olive oil (some)
- 1 teaspoon sea salt
- Pepper
- 1 tbsp sugar (possibly icing sugar)
- 1/2 bunch of thyme (leaves plucked and chopped)

Preparation

1. Wash the vegetables and dry them with kitchen paper. Cut everything into large cubes.

2. Marinate in a bowl with oil, sea salt and sugar. Add the thyme to the vegetables and mix in a bowl.
3. Place the marinated vegetables on the grid insert and cook in the hot air fryer at 180 ° C for 15-18 minutes.
4. Serve sprinkled with fresh herbs.

Crispy spring rolls from the hot air fryer

Ingredients

- 110 g carrots
- 110 g corn
- 110 g peas (frozen)
- 1 tbsp coriander
- 1/4 head of iceberg lettuce
- 1/2 chili peppers
- 1/2 tbsp sesame oil
- 1 tbsp soy sauce
- some leaf spring rolls
- 1 egg

Preparation

1. For crispy spring rolls, first wash the carrots and dice them finely. Drain the corn. Cook the carrots and peas in salted water until they are al dente. In the meantime, wash, dry and finely chop the

coriander. Wash the iceberg lettuce, spin dry and cut into thin strips. Core and finely chop the chilli pepper.
2. Mix the vegetables with the sesame oil, soy sauce, chilli, coriander, lettuce, and season with salt and pepper.
3. Whisk the egg. Put on a sheet of spring roll, brush the egg and place a second sheet on top. Cover with the vegetables and roll up. Brush the ends with egg and press together well. Repeat until the vegetables are used up.
4. Place the spring rolls on the (greased) grill cup and bake in the air fryer at 200 ° C for about 15 minutes. Serve crispy spring rolls immediately.

Red-white-red casserole from the air fryer

- Preparation time 15mins
- Cooking time 30mins
- Servings 4

Ingredients

- 250 g beets
- 250 g potatoes

For the cast:
- 250 ml sour cream
- 3 eggs
- 125 ml whipped cream
- 100 g cheese
- salt
- Pepper (from the mill)
- Culinary herbs

Preparation

1. The red-white-red casserole first cook the beets and potatoes until they are firm to the bite (you can do it the day before).
2. Peel the potatoes and beets and cut into approx. 1 cm thick slices. Alternately place in the (lightly greased) baking tin.
3. Grate the cheese. Mix with all the other ingredients for the glaze and pour over the vegetables.
4. Bake the red-white-red casserole in the hot air fryer at 170 ° C for about 25 minutes.

Sweet potato fries from the air fryer

Ingredients

- 800 g sweet potatoes
- 1 tbsp sesame seeds
- 1/2 tbsp sea salt (coarse)
- some oil

preparation

1. Peel the sweet potatoes and cut them into 1 x 1 cm thick French fries.
2. Toast the sesame without fat until it smells fragrant. Let cool a little and pound with the salt.
3. Bake the sweet potato fries in the hot air fryer with a little oil at 200 ° C for about 10 minutes. Then reduce the temperature to 180 ° C and bake for another 15 minutes.
4. Sprinkle with the sesame and salt mixture and serve immediately.

Spicy puff pastry roses from the hot air fryer

- Cooking time 15 to 30 min
- Servings: 6

Ingredients

- 1 packet of puff pastry
- 1 zucchini
- 150 g soft cheese
- 6 teaspoons parmesan
- salt
- pepper

Preparation

1. For savory puff pastry roses from the hot air fryer, first grate both types of cheese finely. Wash the zucchini, cut off the ends and cut the zucchini in half lengthways. Then cut into very thin slices (semicircles).
2. Roll out the puff pastry and cut lengthways into 6 equal strips. Place the

zucchini slices with the round side up close together at the top of the strips (the zucchini slices should be about halfway on the puff pastry).
3. Sprinkle with the two types of cheese, then season with salt and pepper. Fold the puff pastry strip over the courgette side from below (the courgette's round side should not be covered with puff pastry). Carefully roll the strips into a rose.
4. Grease a muffin tin and put in the savory puff pastry roses from the air fryer. Bake at 200 ° C in the hot air fryer for about 15-20 minutes.

Vegetable nuggets from the air fryer

- Cooking time More than 60 min
- Servings: 4

Ingredients

- 200 g potatoes (floury)
- 300 g vegetables (frozen, mixed, e.g. peas, carrots, corn)
- 1 egg
- 50 grams of flour
- 1 pinch of salt
- 1 pinch of pepper

For the panier:
- 100 g of flour
- 100 g of crumbs
- 2 eggs

Preparation

1. Peel the potatoes and cook in hot water for about 20 minutes. Boil the frozen vegetables with a little water.
2. As soon as the potatoes are done, press them through a potato press or roughly grind them with a kitchen grater. Add the vegetables, egg and flour, season with salt and pepper.
3. Shape into a rectangular mass. Cut rectangular nuggets from the mass.
4. First turn each loaf in flour, pull through the beaten eggs and roll in breadcrumbs.
5. Brush the nuggets with a little oil, bake in the hot air fryer for 15 to 20 minutes at 180 ° C.

Chanterelle goulash from the hot air fryer

- Cooking time 15 to 30 min
- Servings: 4

Ingredients

- 800 g chanterelles
- 50 ml of vegetable oil
- 100 g onions
- 125 ml sour cream
- 10 g paprika powder (noble sweet)
- 3 tbsp vinegar
- 1 teaspoon flour
- salt
- Pepper (from the mill)

Preparation

1. For the chanterelle goulash from the hot air fryer, first clean the chanterelles and cut into bite-sized pieces depending on their size. Peel and dice the onions.

2. Fry the onions with a little oil for 1-2 minutes at 180 ° C in the hot air fryer. Add paprika powder, vinegar, chanterelles, salt and pepper, mix well and cook for another 10-12 minutes until soft.
3. In the meantime, stir the sour cream with the flour until smooth. Stir into the chanterelle goulash from the air fryer and cook for another 5 minutes.

Light potato and zucchini patties from the hot air fryer

Ingredients

- 500 g potatoes (preferably floury, cooked)
- 350 g zucchini
- 300 g cream cheese (low-fat version)
- 1/2 bunch of parsley (fresh)
- 1 pinch of salt
- 1 pinch of pepper
- 1 pinch of nutmeg
- 100 g of flour

For the panier:
- 100 g of flour
- 100 g of crumbs
- 2 eggs
- 2 tbsp oil (for spraying or brushing)

Preparation

1. Wash and roughly grate the zucchini, add a little salt and let stand for a few minutes.
2. In the meantime, peel the potatoes, press them through a potato press, or roughly grind them with a kitchen grater.
3. Squeeze the grated zucchini well with your hands so that any excess water is lost.
4. Wash the parsley and chop the leaves.
5. Mix the potatoes with the grated zucchini and mix in the cream cheese, flour and parsley. Season with salt, pepper and a pinch of nutmeg.
6. Shape the mass into flat patties of the same size.
7. First turn each loaf in flour, pull it through the beaten eggs and finally roll it in breadcrumbs.

Vegetable and oat patties from the hot air fryer

- Cooking time 30 to 60 min
- Servings: 4

Ingredients

- 1 onion
- 1 bell pepper
- 4 potatoes
- 2 carrots
- 1 zucchini
- 200 g breadcrumbs (plus more to roll over)
- 100 g of oatmeal
- 2 eggs
- salt
- pepper
- marjoram
- Caraway seed
- Vegetable oil (for brushing)

Preparation

1. For the vegetable and oat patties, first peel and chop the onion. Wash, core and cut the peppers into small cubes. Peel and grate the potatoes and carrots. Grate the zucchini as well.
2. Mix all the ingredients. Shape patties and roll in breadcrumbs.
3. The vegetable oat patties brush with oil and place in the Airfryer basket and the Air fryer bake at 180 ° C for about 10 minutes. Repeat until all of the patties are done.

Zucchini chips from the air fryer

- Cooking time More than 60 min
- Servings: 4

Ingredients

- 2 zucchini
- 1 clove of garlic
- 30 g parmesan cheese
- 1 tbsp apple cider vinegar
- some salt

Preparation

- For the zucchini chips, do not slice the zucchini too thinly. Peel and squeeze the garlic. Finely grate the parmesan.
- Mix all the ingredients.
- Place the zucchini slices individually on the (greased) grill plate. Bake in the hot air fryer at 160 ° C for 10 minutes until the chips get some colour. Then bake at 110 ° C for about 50 minutes until they are crispy.

- The parmesan shell ensures that the zucchini chips are crispy. Keep looking back and being careful not to burn the zucchini chips. Repeat until all the zucchini slices are used up.
- A variant:
- If you want great, crispy crisps through and through, and have a little patience, let the zucchini slices bake for 10 minutes at 160 ° C and then for 5 hours at only 70 ° C.
- It is worth it!

Zucchini and feta casserole from the hot air fryer

- Cooking time 30 to 60 min
- Servings: 2

Ingredients

- 500 g zucchini
- 100 g feta
- 2 eggs
- 1 tbsp milk
- salt
- Pepper (from the mill)
- 1 1/2 tbsp olive oil

Preparation

1. Wash the zucchini and grate roughly. Squeeze out very well so that as little liquid as possible remains.
2. Whisk the eggs with the milk. Mix the crumbled feta with the remaining ingredients.

3. Pour into the greased baking pan and pour the egg-milk mixture over it.
4. Bake the casserole in the hot air fryer at 180 ° C for about 30-35 minutes.

Corn skewers from the air fryer

Ingredients

- 3 ears of corn
- some corn oil
- some butter
- salt
- Skewers (for the air fryer)

Preparation

1. First, the corn skewers from the hot air fryer clean the corn on the cob and cut into slices about 2-2 1/2 cm thick. Put them on the skewers with a little space. Brush with oil. Grill at around 180 ° C for 10-15 minutes in the hot air fryer.
2. In the meantime, melt the butter. Brush the finished corn skewers from the hot air fryer with butter and sprinkle with salt.

Side Dish

Air Fryer corn on The Cob

- Cooking time 30 to 60 min
- servings 4

Ingredients

- 3 ear cups and silk removed
- 1 tbsp of olive oil and a little more to brush the corn
- 1 tbsp lime juice
- 1/4 tsp paprika
- 1 tbsp parmesan and a little more to garnish
- Salt and pepper
- 1 tablespoon finely chopped parsley

Preparation

1. Preheat the oven to 390F (takes about 2-3minutes at the mine)
2. Gently apply oil on the corn's surface and place it in an air pan. Cook for some minutes
3. turn the corn and cook for another 3-5 minutes.
4. Mix olive oil, lemon juice, paprika, Parmesan cheese, salt and pepper in a bowl. and mix them
5. If using corn, scrub regularly with a mixture of oil and lemon.
6. At the end, sprinkle with grated Parmesan cheese and a little fresh parsley. Provide warm service

Air Fryer Potato Latkes

- Cooking time 30 mins
- servings 4

Ingredients

- 2 large Russet potatoes, peeled and grated
- 1 medium sized white onion, grated
- 1/2 cup almond flour.
- 2 large eggs
- 1 teaspoon salt
- Ground black pepper to taste
- Spray for cooking
- Garlic flavoured

Preparation

1. Put the grated potatoes and onions into a peanut milk bag, a cloth or kitchen cloth and squeeze out all the water. Add to a large mixing bowl.

2. Add the remaining ingredients to the mixing bowl. Stir until combined.
3. Use 1/4 scoop. Put the potato mixture in a measuring cup and mix by hand to make a pancake mold. (Will be almost the size of a hand)
4. Spray the skillet on the pan. Place the rake in one layer of the air basket (the amount depends on the basket size). Avoid overlapping.
5. Fry for 15 minutes at 400 ° F (longer if you want crispy). He turns halfway.
6. Remove from the deep fryer and repeat steps 3-5 until charging is complete.
7. Choose garlic and non-fat Greek yogurt to decorate your favorite toppings and bath sauce!

Sampan Copycat: Air Fried Brussels Sprouts

- Cooking time 30 to 60 min
- servings 2

Ingredients

- 1 pound Brussels sprouts, trimmed tips, outer leaves removed and divided in half
- 2 tablespoons fish sauce; we used the Extra Boat Vietnamese red fish sauce.
- 2 tablespoons of pure maple syrup
- 1 tablespoon of coconut amino acids (or soy sauce with reduced sodium content)
- 1 tbsp Sriracha (or less if you don't like spicy)
- 1 garlic clove, chopped
- extra virgin olive oil spray

Preparation

1. Add one layer of the prepared Brussels sprouts to the fried basket and lightly spray with olive oil spray.
2. Fry in Brussels for 20 minutes at 400°F (trust us). Throw every 5 minutes.
3. When you have about 5-10 minutes in Brussels, add the remaining ingredients to a small pan and bring to a boil. When boiling, boil the heat. Wait for the sauce to decrease and thicken for about 5 minutes.
4. Add fried Brussels to a large mixing bowl. Pour the sauce into Brussels and toss until a uniform coating is obtained.

Air-Fried Pickles with Chipotle Dipping Sauce

- Cooking time 15-30 min
- servings 4

Ingredients

- 1 cup hamburger dill pickle chips
- 3/4 cup panko
- 1/4 cup almond flour
- 2 eggs
- salt and pepper, to taste
- cooking spray

For the chipotle dipping sauce:
- 1 chipotle pepper + 1 tsp adobo sauce
- 1/2 cup plain non-fat Greek yogurt
- 1/4 tsp cumin
- 1/4 tsp salt

Preparation

1. Combine ingredients for the dipping sauce in a blender of a food processor and blend until combined. Set aside or chill until ready to serve.
2. Preheat air fryer to 400°F.
3. Lay pickles out on a dry surface and pat with paper towels to dry.
4. Set up your dredging station by placing almond flour in a small bowl, eggs in another small bowl (whisking until scrambled), panko, salt and pepper in another bowl (mixing until combined).
5. One at a time, coat pickle chips in almond flour, egg, and panko, in that order, until all pickle chips are evenly coated.
6. Place half of the pickles in a single layer in the basket of your air fryer and lightly spray with cooking spray. Cook for 8 minutes, flipping halfway through. Repeat this step with the remaining pickles. Serve with dipping sauce.

Air Fryer Avocado Fries + Sriracha Ketchup

- preparation time 60 min
- servings 4

Ingredient

- Avocado in 1
- 1/4 cup seasoned bread crumbs
- 2 teaspoons pecorino romano cheese
- 1 egg
- Cooking spray
- salt, taste
- For Sriracha Ketchup:
- 2 tablespoons ketchup. We used Annie's homemade organic ketchup.
- 2 teaspoons Sriracha

Preparation

1. Mix ketchup and sriracha until completely combined. I'll save it.
2. Preheat the air fryer to 400 ° F.

3. Set up the dr station with breadcrumbs and cheese in a small bowl. Scrambled eggs in another small bowl.
4. Slice the avocado into about 8-10 thin strips.
5. Soak avocado in eggs one at a time and mix with bread crumbs. Repeat this until all avocado slices are coated.
6. Put half of the avocado in the air fryer basket and lightly spray with cooking spray. Turn it over and cook for 8 minutes. Repeat this procedure for the remaining avocado fly.
7. Lightly season the avocado with salt and eat with shiracha ketchup.

Air Fryer Buffalo Turkey Meatball

Ingredients

- 1 lb. 93% lean ground turkey (or ground chicken)
- 2 tbsp coconut flour
- 1 egg
- 1/4 cup diced carrots
- 1/4 cup diced celery
- 2 scallions, chopped
- 1 clove garlic
- salt and pepper, to taste
- cooking spray

For the sauce:
- 2 tbsp ghee; we used Himalayan Pink Salt Grass-Fed Ghee Butter by 4th & Heart.
- 1/3 cup hot sauce; our go-to is Frank's.

Preparation

1. Spray the air fryer basket with cooking spray and preheat the air fryer to 400 ° F.
2. Place the meatball ingredients in a large bowl and mix by hand until they are fully joined. Form meatballs into approximately 1.5-inch balls. You need to get about 20 meatballs.
3. Cook the meatballs for 12 minutes with a preheated air fryer and rotate them halfway. Note: The meatballs must be cooked in two portions. Avoid overcrowding the air fryer.
4. When the second batch of meatballs is almost finished, fry in a small pan over medium heat and add ghee and hot sauce. When the ghee melts, whisk and mix. Removed from the heat.
    a. When meatballs are finished frying, toss in the sauce.
5. HACK: I like to put the meatballs in a Tupperware, pour the sauce over the meatballs, put the lid on tightly and shake to ensure even coating.

6. Garnish with toppings of your choice: blue cheese crumbles, scallions, etc., and serve!

Raclette In the Air fryer

- Cooking time 15 to 30 min
- servings 4

Ingredient

- 1 kg big potatoes, cooked
- 500g raclette cheese
- 200 g mushrooms
- 2 Red onions
- 2 paprika
- 200 g Cherry tomatoes
- Herb quark
- Something Bread to serve
- Salt and pepper

Preparation

1. Halve the potatoes and hollow them out with a spoon (the potato interior can be used as a side dish for a potato salad, for example). Dice the onions, peppers and mushrooms and fill them into bowls. Halve the cherry tomatoes and cut the raclette cheese so that one slice fits on one potato half.
2. Fill the potato halves with some vegetables and then cover with a cheese slice. Cook in the Air fryer at 180 ° C for 6-8 minutes until the cheese has melted. Depending on how crusty you like your cheese, you can cook the potatoes after 6 minutes again for 2 minutes at 200 ° C.
3. Season with salt and pepper and serve with bread, herb quark and your favourite raclette side dishes.

Rack of Lamb with Herb Crust from The Air fryer

- Cooking time 30 to 60 min
- servings 8

Ingredient

- 6 Rack of lamb, pre-cut
- 1 tbsp   olive oil
- 1 clove of garlic
- salt and pepper
- 1 tbsp   fresh rosemary, finely chopped
- 1 tbsp dried thyme
- 40g Butter, melted
- 20g Panko breadcrumbs
- 50g Almonds, chopped
- salt and pepper

For the side dishes

- 500g beetroot, cooked (+ 3 tbsp beetroot juice)
- 800g potatoes

- 50g butter
- salt and pepper
- 1 prs nutmeg
- 3 tbsp grated Parmesan
- fresh parsley, chopped

Preparation

1. Boil water in a large pot. Peel the potatoes and cook with the beetroot for about 30 minutes until the potatoes are tender. Add the butter and work with a potato masher until the puree is creamy. Season with nutmeg, salt and pepper.
2. Now marinate the rack of lamb. Brush with olive oil, season with salt and pepper and sprinkle with garlic. To prepare the herb breadcrumbs: mix the butter, rosemary, thyme, panko breadcrumbs, salt and pepper and spread on the meat. Place on the Air fryer's grill pan and cook at 200 ° C for 10 minutes.

3. Melt the Parmesan in the Air fryer baking pan and allow to cool. Break into small pieces.
4. Arrange some puree on a plate and lay the meat on it. Then garnish with Parmesan asparagus and fresh parsley.

Spicy Carrots from The Air fryer

- Cooking time 15 to 30 min
- servings 2

Ingredient

- 500g carrots
- ½ Lemon, juice and peel
- 1 Garlic clove, finely chopped
- 2 tbsp   olive oil
- 1 teaspoon   Ras el-Hanout
- 1 prs Harissa
- salt and pepper
- 70g dried cranberries
- 30g planed almonds
- Spring onions for garnish
- Lemon slices to serve

Preparation

1. Peel and halve the carrots. Mix with olive oil, garlic clove, Ras el-Hanout, Harissa, lemon juice, peel, salt, and pepper. Cook in the Air fryer at 180 ° C for 15 minutes.
2. Mix with cranberries and almonds. Finally serve with a little chopped spring onion and lemon wedges.

COQ Au Vin from The Air fryer

Ingredient

- 3 shallots
- 1 spring onion
- carrots
- 150ml   chicken stock
- 150ml   strong red wine
- 1 teaspoon   Paprika powder (Rosenschaft & Edelsüß)
- 2 Garlic cloves
- about 300g   Chicken (fillet or leg)
- something   Pepper salt
- something   thyme
- 1-2 Branches of fresh rosemary
- 1 Lemon peel (abrasion)
- 3 tbsp   olive oil

Preparation

1. For the marinade mince a carrot, spring onion, shallot and garlic. Put in a bowl and add the wine, chicken stock, paprika, thyme and rosemary (fresh if possible) and the lemon. Mix with the chicken and set aside for at least 30 minutes.
2. Chop the remaining carrots, shallots and garlic and sauté for 5 minutes at 180 ° C in the Air fryer's baking dish with a little olive oil.
3. Then put the chicken drumsticks on top and put the bowl's contents in the baking dish. Stir for 30 minutes at 140 ° C. If chicken drumsticks are used, turn them once after 15 minutes.
4. Serve on a deep plate. Potato dumplings or baked potatoes are excellent as a side dish. The latter can simply be prepared in the Air fryer: pour a little water into the soil and cook at 180 ° C for 30 minutes.

Air Fryer Corn on The Cob

- Preparation time 5mins
- Cooking time 10mins
- Servings 2

Ingredients

- 3 ear cups and silk removed
- 1 tbsp of olive oil and a little more to brush the corn
- 1 tbsp lime juice
- 1/4 tsp paprika
- 1 tbsp parmesan and a little more to garnish
- Salt and pepper
- 1 tablespoon finely chopped parsley

Preparation

1. Preheat the oven to 390F (takes about 2-3minutes at the mine)

2. Gently apply oil on the corn's surface and place it in an air pan. Cook for some minutes
3. turn the corn and cook for another 3-5 minutes.
4. Mix olive oil, lemon juice, paprika, Parmesan cheese, salt and pepper in a bowl. and mix them
5. If using corn, scrub regularly with a mixture of oil and lemon.
6. At the end, sprinkle with grated Parmesan cheese and a little fresh parsley. Provide warm service

Egg Salad

- Cooking time More than 60 min
- servings 4

Ingredients

- 8 eggs (hard-boiled)
- 150 g pineapple
- 150 g mayonnaise
- 2 tbsp whipped cream
- 1 tbsp curry (milder)
- 1 pinch of cayenne pepper
- salt
- 1 pinch of sugar
- Worcester sauce (a few drops)
- 2 teaspoons sweet chili sauce

Preparation

1. For the egg salad, cut the eggs in half and into wedges. Cut the pineapple into small cubes and place everything in a bowl.
2. The dressing mix the mayonnaise with the whipped cream and the spices and season

with the sauces to taste. Pour over the salad and fold in carefully. Let the egg salad steep in the refrigerator.

Potato and rocket salad

- Preparation time 15mins
- Cooking time 30mins
- Servings 4

Ingredients

- 800 g potatoes (greasy and cooked)
- 100 g rocket
- 1 teaspoon mustard
- 150 g onions (finely chopped)
- 100 ml pumpkin seed oil
- 100 ml white wine vinegar
- 200 ml beef soup (warm)
- salt
- pepper
- sugar

Preparation

1. For the potato and rocket salad the mustard with the pumpkin seed oil, vinegar, warm beef soup, salt, pepper, and

a little sugar. Slice the still-warm potatoes into leaves and add a little salt.
2. Cut the rocket and mix with the finely chopped onions in the marinade. Then mix with the potatoes.

Potato and celery puree

- preparation time 15mins
- cooking time 30mins
- servings 4

Ingredients
- 300 g celery
- 200 g potatoes (up to 300 g, floury)
- some milk (or whipped cream)
- 50 g butter (up to 80 g)
- salt
- Pepper (white, from the mill)

Preparation
1. For the potato-celery puree, peel the celery and potatoes, quarter them and cook in salted water mixed with a little milk until soft. Strain and mash with a potato masher or puree briefly.
2. Season the potato and celery puree with salt and a little white pepper, and round off the taste with milk or cream and butter.

Semolina dumplings

- Cooking time More than 60 min
- servings 6

ingredients

- 40 g white bread, debarked
- 1/4 l milk
- 35 g butter
- 75 g semolina
- 1 egg
- Salt, nutmeg

Preparation

1. For the semolina dumplings, dice white bread. Bring the milk and butter to the boil, stir in the semolina and cook until the semolina is soft. Let the semolina cool over. Mix in egg and white bread cubes, season.

2. Let the mixture rest for 1 hour. Portion dumplings to 50 g each, shape and simmer for 10 minutes.

Croquettes from the air fryer

- preparation time 5mins
- cooking time 15mins
- servings 2

Ingredients

- 8-10 croquettes (frozen)
- 1 tbsp olive oil

Preparation

1. For the croquettes from the air fryer, put 1 tablespoon of olive oil in a soup plate and toss the frozen croquettes in it.
2. Bake in the air fryer at 200 ° C for 6 minutes

Pumpkin wedges from the air fryer

- preparation time 15mins
- cooking time 30mins
- servings 4

ingredients

- 1 pc. Pumpkin (Hokaido)
- 3-4 tbsp oil
- Spicy Spice

Preparation

1. For the pumpkin wedges from the air fryer, cut the pumpkin into quarters, remove the seeds and then cut into thin wedges.
2. Mix the oil with the spice and mix in a bowl with the pumpkin wedges.
3. Bake in the hot air fryer at 180 ° C for about 10 minutes, take the basket out of the deep fryer, carefully mix the pumpkin pieces and then bake for about 8 minutes at 200 ° C.

Corn skewers from the air fryer

- preparation time 5mins
- cooking time 15mins
- servings 4

Ingredients

- 3 ears of corn
- some corn oil
- some butter
- salt
- Skewers (for the air fryer)

Preparation

1. First, the corn skewers from the hot air fryer clean the corn on the cob and cut into slices about 2-2 1/2 cm thick. Put them on the skewers with a little space. Brush with oil.
2. Grill at around 180 ° C for 10-15 minutes in the hot air fryer.

3. In the meantime, melt the butter. Brush the finished corn skewers from the hot air fryer with butter and sprinkle with salt.

DESSERT, SWEETS AND SNACKS

Fried Bananas S'mores

Ingredients

- 4 bananas
- 3 tablespoons mini half-sweet pieces of chocolate
- 3 tablespoons of mini peanut butter chips
- 3 tablespoons of mini marshmallows
- 3 Tablespoons of Graham Cracker Muesli

Preparation

1. Preheat the air fryer to 400°F.
2. Slice the unpeeled bananas lengthwise along the inside of the curve, but do not cut through the bottom of the shell. Open the banana lightly to form a bag.

3. Fill each bag with chocolate chips, peanut butter pieces and marshmallows. Add Graham Cracker Muesli to the filling.
4. Place the bananas in the air frying basket and place them on top of each other to keep them upright with the filling up. Fry for 6 minutes in the air or until the banana feels soft, the skin is blackened and the chocolate and marshmallows are melted and roasted.
5. Let it cool for a few minutes and then simply serve it with a spoon to spoon out the filling.

Air fryer Apple Pie

- Cooking time 60 min
- servings 4

Ingredient

- 1 Pillsbury refrigerator puff pastry
- Baking spray
- 1 big chopped apple
- 2 teaspoons of lemon juice
- 1 tablespoon cinnamon
- 2 tablespoons sugar
- 1/2 teaspoon vanilla essence
- 1 tablespoon butter
- 1 beaten egg
- 1 tablespoon sugar

Preparation

1. Thaw the ready-made pie skin according to the package instructions.

2. While preparing the pie, preheat Air fryer to the highest degree.
3. Using a smaller baking tin, cut one crust 1/3 inch larger than the tin and the second crust slightly smaller than the baking tin. You may need to rotate the crust a little with a rolling pin to stretch the pie crust. Save the smaller ones.
4. Spray on baking cans with baking spray and place large cut crust on the baking pan. I'll save it.
5. In a small bowl, add chopped apple, lemon juice, cinnamon, sugar, and vanilla essence. Mix and mix.
6. Pour apples into the baking pan with puff pastry.
7. Top apple with butter.
8. Place the second puff pastry on top of the apple and pick the end. Make some slits at the top of the dough.
9. Spread the beaten egg on top of the crust and sprinkle the raw sugar on top of the egg mixture.
10. Place the pie in the Air Fryer basket.

11. Set a timer for 30 minutes at 320 degrees

Roasted Apples in Jocca Oil-Free Fryer

Ingredients

- 4 portions
- 4 apples
- 4 ctas dulce de leche
- ice cream to serve and mint to serve

Preparation

1. We wash the apples and sprig we take out a large part of the applesauce.
2. We put a can of dulce de leche (you can also put sugar and a little muscatel).
3. We put them in the basket and program 180° 18 minutes when the time ends, see if they are ready, and withdraw. If you see that it is missing a little, we leave them 2 more minutes.

4. Let cool and serve with a lemon ice cream and mint leaves. A healthy, quick and delicious rich dessert.

Baked Apple from The Air fryer

Ingredient

- 4 apples
- 30g raisins
- 40g chopped hazelnuts
- 2 tbsp honey
- 1/2 tsp cinnamon
- vanilla extract

Preparation

1. Core the apples. Mix raisins, hazelnuts, honey, cinnamon and vanilla extract fill the apples with the mass.
2. At 180 ° C for 10 minutes in the air fryer.

Crispy baked apple with rum and raisins

Ingredients

- 4 apples
- 4 tbsp raisins
- 4 tbsp rum
- 30 g butter
- 3 tbsp oatmeal
- 5 tbsp granulated sugar
- 5 tbsp whipped cream

Preparation

1. The crispy baked apple with rum raisins , let the raisins steep in the rum for one to two hours. Cut the lid off the apples and remove the core. Cut off the lower part of the apple so that it can stand firmly in place.

2. Melt the butter in a pan and sprinkle with the oatmeal and sugar. Lightly toast the oat flakes or caramelize the sugar while stirring constantly. Then remove the mixture from the stove and stir in the whipped cream. Finally, mix in the marinated raisins.
3. Grease an ovenproof dish with butter and sprinkle with breadcrumbs. Insert the apples, fill with the mixture and put the lid back on.
4. Bake the crispy baked apple with rum and raisins in the oven preheated to 220 ° C for about 30 minutes.

Strawberry muffins

Ingredients

- 280 g flour
- 200 g of sugar
- 2 teaspoons of baking powder
- 1/2 teaspoon baking soda
- 1 pc egg
- 120 ml of oil
- 1/4 l buttermilk
- 250 g strawberries
- 1 teaspoon cinnamon

Preparation

1. For the strawberry muffins, stir the egg with the sugar until frothy. Stir in the oil and buttermilk and continue to beat until frothy. Sift the baking powder and baking soda into the flour and add the cinnamon.

2. Carefully fold the flour mixture into the egg-sugar mixture. Cut the strawberries into small pieces and mix with the batter. Now pour the mixture immediately into the muffin tray and bake with hot air at 160 degrees on the middle rack for about 20 minutes.
3. Let the strawberry muffins cool and serve.

Plantain Chips

Ingredients

- 1000 g plantain (green)
- 500 ml of peanut oil
- Salt

Preparation

1. First, plantain chips remove the skin from the plantain and cut across into 10-12 oblong slices. Rub with a little bit of salt. Heat the oil and fry the banana pieces until golden brown on both sides.
2. Remove the banana pieces and drain them on a paper towel. The plantain chips nibble still warm.

Bruschette with tomato topping

- preparation time 15mins
- cooking time 30mins
- servings 8

Ingredients

- 8 slices of bruschettas (or fluffy white bread)
- 2 pieces of meat tomatoes (pitted)
- 2 cloves of garlic (pressed)
- 1 tbsp basil leaves
- 2 tbsp olive oil
- salt
- Pepper (freshly ground)

Preparation

1. For the bruschetta with tomato topping, mix all the ingredients well and season. Brown the bread slices in the oven preheated to 250 ° C for about 4 minutes. Spread the tomato topping and serve immediately.

Sandwich cake

Ingredients

- 12 slice (s) of toast
- 250 g low-fat curd
- 350 g mayonnaise
- 300 ml whipped cream
- 1 can (s) of tuna
- 300 g ham
- 3 eggs (hard-boiled)
- Dill (for sprinkling)

Preparation

1. For the sandwich cake, whip the whipped cream until stiff and mix it with the curd and mayonnaise. Divide into three bowls.
2. Mix part of the mixture with tuna and one with ham. Save the rest of the mixture to finish off the sandwich cake.

Baked tuna breads

Ingredients

- 4 slice (s) bread (dark)
- 1 can (s) of tuna (natural)
- 1 onion (peeled and chopped)
- 125 ml yoghurt (1%)
- 120 g cheese (grated, light)
- chives
- salt
- pepper

Preparation

1. Mix the tuna with the onion, yoghurt, cheese, chives, salt and pepper.
2. Spread the mixture on the bread.
3. Baked in the oven at 200 ° C.

Fried onion

- Preparation time 15mins
- Cooking time 30mins
- Servings 4

Ingredients

- 2 onions (large)
- Flour
- Vegetable oil
- Paprika powder (noble sweet; optional)

Preparation

1. For the fried onions, first, peel the onions and cut into fine rings. Push apart.
2. Put the flour on a flat plate (and mix with the paprika powder to taste). Turn the onion rings in it.
3. Heat enough oil in a pan. Knock off the onion rings a little and then fry them in portions in hot oil until crispy. Take out the fried onion and drain on a kitchen roll.

Minced patties

- Preparation time 15mins
- Cooking time 30mins
- Servings 4

Ingredients

- 500 g minced meat (mixed)
- 2 rolls
- 30 g butter
- 50 g onions (chopped)
- 1/2 bunch of parsley (chopped)
- 2 eggs
- 30 g crumbs
- salt
- pepper
- 200 g of oil
- 50 g flour

Preparation

1. Soak the rolls, press them out and knead with the minced meat, butter, onions, parsley, eggs, breadcrumbs, salt, pepper and marjoram to a homogeneous mass.
2. Shape patties with wet hands, turn in flour and slowly fry in hot fat until crispy.
3. Arrange and serve the minced patties.

Breaded zucchini

- Preparation time 15mins
- Cooking time 30mins

Ingredients

- 2 zucchinis (unpeeled)
- egg (whisked)
- 1 tbsp parsley (smooth, chopped)
- 1 tbsp breadcrumbs
- tbsp olive oil
- 1 tbsp lemon (juice)
- salt
- Pepper (freshly ground)

Preparation

1. Cut the zucchini into slices, season the zucchini slices with salt and pepper.
2. Mix the egg and parsley. Dip the zucchini slices in it, then turn in breadcrumbs.
3. Fry until golden brown in hot oil. Drain on kitchen paper and drizzle with lemon juice.

Air Fryer Sweet Potato Tots

Ingredients

- 2 small (14 oz. total) sweet potatoes, peeled
- tablespoon potato starch
- 1/8 teaspoon garlic powder
- 1 1/4 teaspoons kosher salt, divided
- 3/4 cup no-salt-added ketchup
- Cooking spray

Preparation

1. Bring a medium pot of water to a boil over high heat. Add potatoes, and cook until just fork tender, about 15 minutes. Transfer potatoes to a plate to cool, about 15 minutes.

2. Working over a medium bowl, grate potatoes using the large holes of a box grater. Gently toss with potato starch, garlic powder and 1 teaspoon salt. Shape mixture into about 24 (1-inch) tot-shaped cylinders.

3. Lightly coat air fryer basket with cooking spray. Place 1/2 of tots (about 12) in single layer in the basket, and spray with cooking spray. Cook at 400°F until lightly browned, 12 to 14 minutes, turning tots halfway through cook time. Remove from fry basket and sprinkle with 1/8 teaspoon salt. Repeat with remaining tots and salt. Serve immediately with ketchup.

Air Fryer Banana Bread

Ingredients

- 3/4 cup (3 oz.) white-whole wheat flour
- teaspoon cinnamon
- 1/2 teaspoon Kosher salt
- 1/4 teaspoon Baking soda 2 medium (12 oz. total) ripe bananas,
- mashed (about 3/4 cup) 2 large eggs,
- lightly beaten 1/2 cup granulated sugar
- 1/3 cup plain nonfat yogurt 2 tablespoons vegetable oil
- teaspoon Vanilla extract 2 tablespoons (3/4 oz.) toasted walnuts, roughly

Preparation

1. Line the bottom of a 6-inch round cake pan with parchment paper; lightly coat pan with cooking spray. Whisk together flour, cinnamon, salt and baking soda in a medium bowl; set aside.

2. In separate medium bowl, whisk together mashed bananas, eggs, sugar, yogurt, oil and vanilla. Gently stir wet ingredients into flour mixture until well combined. Pour batter into prepared pan and sprinkle with walnuts.

3. Heat a 5.3-qt air fryer to 310°F and then place pan in air fryer and cook until browned and a wooden pick inserted in the middle comes out clean, 30 to 35 minutes, turning pan halfway through cook time. Transfer bread to a wire rack to cool in pan for 15 minutes before turning out and slicing.

Air Fryer Avocado Fries

Ingredients

- 1/2 cup (about 2 1/8 oz.) all-purpose flour
- 1/2 teaspoons black pepper
- large eggs 1 tablespoon water
- 1/2 cup panko (Japanese-style breadcrumbs)
- avocados, cut into 8 wedges each
- Cooking spray
- 1/4 teaspoon kosher salt
- 1/4 cup no-salt-added ketchup
- 2 tablespoons canola mayonnaise
- 1 tablespoon apple cider vinegar
- 1 tablespoon Sriracha chili sauce

Preparation

1. Stir together flour and pepper in a shallow dish. Lightly beat eggs and water in a second shallow dish. Place panko in a third shallow dish. Dredge avocado wedges in flour, shaking off excess. Dip in egg mixture, allowing any excess to drip off. Dredge in panko, pressing to adhere. Coat avocado wedges well with cooking spray.

2. Place avocado wedges in air fryer basket, and cook at 400°F until golden, 7 to 8 minutes, turning avocado wedges over halfway through cooking. Remove from air fryer; sprinkle with salt.

3. While avocado wedges cook, whisk together ketchup, mayonnaise, vinegar, and Sriracha in a small bowl. To serve, place 4 avocado fries on each plate with 2 tablespoons sauce.

Air Fryer Churros With Chocolate Sauce

Ingredients

- 1/2 cup water
- 1/4 teaspoon kosher salt
- 1/4 cup , plus 2 Tbsp. unsalted butter, divided
- 1/2 cup (about 2 1/8 oz.) all-purpose flour
- 2 large eggs
- 1/3 cup granulated sugar
- 2 teaspoons ground cinnamon
- 4 ounces bittersweet baking chocolate, finely chopped
- 3 tablespoons heavy cream
- 2 tablespoons vanilla kefir

Preparation

1. Bring water, salt, and 1/4 cup of the butter to a boil in a small saucepan over medium-high. Reduce heat to medium-low; add flour, and stir vigorously with a wooden spoon until dough is smooth, about 30 seconds. Continue cooking, stirring constantly, until dough begins to pull away from sides of pan and a film forms on bottom of pan, 2 to 3 minutes. Transfer dough to a medium bowl. Stir constantly until slightly cooled, about 1 minute. Add eggs, 1 at a time, stirring constantly until completely smooth after each addition. Transfer mixture to a piping bag fitted with a medium star tip. Chill 30 minutes.
2. Pipe 6 (3-inch long) pieces in single layer in air fryer basket. Cook at 380°F until golden, about 10

minutes. Repeat with remaining dough.

3. Stir together sugar and cinnamon in a medium bowl. Brush cooked churros with remaining 2 tablespoons melted butter, and roll in sugar mixture to coat.

4. Place chocolate and cream in a small microwavable bowl. Microwave on HIGH until melted and smooth, about 30 seconds, stirring after 15 seconds. Stir in kefir. Serve churros with chocolate sauce.

Air Fryer Southern Style Catfish With Green Beans

Ingredients

- 12 ounces fresh green beans, trimmed
- Cooking spray
- teaspoon light brown sugar
- 1/2 teaspoon crushed red pepper (optional)
- 3/8 teaspoon kosher salt, divided
- Unit (6-oz.) catfish fillets
- 1/4 cup all-purpose flour
- 1 large egg, lightly beaten
- 1/3 cup panko (Japanese-style breadcrumbs)
- 1/4 teaspoon black pepper
- tablespoons mayonnaise
- 1 1/2 teaspoons finely chopped fresh dill
- 3/4 teaspoon dill pickle relish
- 1/2 teaspoon apple cider vinegar

- 1/8 teaspoon granulated sugar Lemon wedges

Preparation

1. Place green beans in a medium bowl, and spray liberally with cooking spray. Sprinkle with brown sugar, crushed red pepper (if using), and 1/8 teaspoon of the salt. Place in air fryer basket, and cook at 400°F until well browned and tender, about 12 minutes. Transfer to a bowl; cover with aluminum foil to keep warm.

2. Meanwhile, toss catfish in flour to coat, shaking excess from fish. Dip pieces, 1 at a time, in egg to coat, then sprinkle with panko, pressing to coat evenly on all sides. Place

3. fish in air fryer basket; spray with cooking spray. Cook at 400°F until browned and cooked through, about 8 minutes.

Sprinkle tops evenly with pepper and remaining 1/4 teaspoon salt.

4. While fish is cooking, whisk together mayonnaise, dill, relish, vinegar, and sugar in a small bowl. Serve fish and green beans with tartar sauce and lemon wedges.

Air Fryer Strawberry Pop Tarts

Ingredients

- 8 ounces quartered strawberries (about 1 3/4 cups)
- 1/4 cup granulated sugar
- 1/2 (14.1-oz.) pkg. refrigerated piecrusts
- Cooking spray
- 1/2 cup (about 2 oz.) powdered sugar
- 1/2 teaspoons fresh lemon juice (from 1 lemon)
- 1/2 ounce rainbow candy sprinkles (about 1 Tbsp.)

Preparation

1. Stir together strawberries and granulated sugar in medium microwavable bowl. Let stand 15 minutes, stirring occasionally. Microwave on HIGH until shiny and reduced, about 10 minutes, stirring

halfway through cooking. Cool completely, about 30 minutes.
2. Roll pie crust into a 12-inch circle on a lightly floured surface. Cut dough into 12 (2 1/2- x 3-inch) rectangles, rerolling scraps, if needed. Spoon about 2 teaspoons strawberry mixture into center of 6 of the dough rectangles, leaving a 1/2-inch border. Brushes edges of filled dough rectangles with water; top with remaining dough rectangles, pressing edges with a fork to seal. Coat tarts well with cooking spray.
3. Place 3 tarts in single layer in air fryer basket, and cook at 350°F until golden brown, about 10 minutes. Repeat with remaining tarts. Place on a wire rack to cool completely, about 30 minutes.
4. Whisk together powdered sugar and lemon juice in a small bowl until smooth. Spoon glaze over cooled tarts, and sprinkle evenly with candy sprinkles.

Air Fryer Empanadas

Ingredients

- tablespoon olive oil
- ounces (85/15) lean ground beef
- 1/4 cup finely chopped white onion
- ounces finely chopped cremini mushrooms
- 2 teaspoons finely chopped garlic
- 6 pitted green olives, chopped
- 1/4 teaspoon paprika
- 1/4 teaspoon ground cumin
- 1/8 teaspoon ground cinnamon
- 1/2 cup chopped tomatoes
- 8 square gyoza wrappers
- 1 large egg, lightly beaten

Preparation

1. Heat oil in a medium skillet over medium-high. Add beef and onion; cook, stirring to crumble, until starting to brown, 3 minutes. Add mushrooms; cook, stirring occasionally, until mushrooms are starting to brown, 6 minutes. Add garlic, olives, paprika, cumin, and cinnamon; cook until mushrooms are very tender and have released most of their liquid, 3 minutes. Stir in tomatoes, and cook 1 minute, stirring occasionally. Transfer filling to a bowl, and let cool 5 minutes.

2. Arrange 4 gyoza wrappers on work surface. Place about 1 1/2 tablespoons filling in center of each wrapper. Brush edges of wrappers with egg; fold wrappers over, pinching edges to seal. Repeat

process with remaining wrappers and filling.

3. Place 4 empanadas in single layer in air fryer basket, and cook at 400°F until nicely browned, 7 minutes. Repeat with remaining empanadas.

Air-Fried Peach Hand Pies

Ingredients

2 (5-oz.) fresh peaches, peeled and chopped

1 tablespoon fresh lemon juice (from 1 lemon)

3 tablespoons granulated sugar

1 teaspoon vanilla extract

1/4 teaspoon table salt

1 teaspoon cornstarch

1 (14.1-oz.) pkg. refrigerated piecrusts

Cooking spray

Preparation

1. Stir together peaches, lemon juice, sugar, vanilla, and salt a in medium bowl. Let stand 15 minutes, stirring occasionally. Drain peaches, reserving 1 tablespoon liquid. Whisk

cornstarch into reserved liquid; stir into drained peaches.

2. Cut piecrusts into 8 (4-inch) circles. Place about 1 tablespoon filling in center of each circle. Brush edges of dough with water; fold dough over filling to form half-moons. Crimp edges with a fork to seal; cut 3 small slits in top of pies. Coat pies well with cooking spray.

3. Place 3 pies in single layer in air fryer basket, and cook at 350°F until golden brown, 12 to 14 minutes. Repeat with remaining pies.

Mexican-Style Air-Fried Corn

Ingredients

- 4 ears fresh corn (about 1 1/2 lb.), shucked
- Cooking spray
- 1/2 tablespoons unsalted butter
- teaspoons chopped garlic
- teaspoon lime zest plus 1 Tbsp. fresh juice (from 1 lime)
- 1/2 teaspoon kosher salt
- 1/2 teaspoon black pepper
- tablespoons chopped fresh cilantro

Preparation

1. Lightly coat corn with cooking spray, and place in a single layer in air fryer basket. Cook at 400°F until tender and slightly charred, 14 minutes, turning corn over halfway through cooking.

2. Meanwhile, stir together butter, garlic, lime zest, and lime juice in a small microwavable bowl. Microwave on HIGH until butter is melted and garlic is fragrant, about 30 seconds. Place corn on a platter and pour over butter mixture. Sprinkle with salt, pepper, and cilantro. Serve immediately.

Air-Fried Whole-Wheat Pita Pizzas

Ingredients

- 1/4 cup lower-sodium marinara sauce
- 2 whole-wheat pita rounds
- cup baby spinach leaves (1 oz.)
- 1 small plum tomato, cut into 8 slices
- 1 small garlic clove, thinly sliced
- 1 ounce pre-shredded part-skim mozzarella cheese (about 1/4 cup)
- 1/4 ounce shaved Parmigiano-Reggiano cheese (about 1 Tbsp.)

Preparation

1. Spread marinara sauce evenly over 1 side of each pita bread. Top with half

each of the spinach leaves, tomato slices, garlic, and cheeses.

2. Place 1 pita in air fryer basket, and cook at 350°F until cheese is melted and pita is crisp, 4 to 5 minutes. Repeat with remaining pita.

Air-Fried Coconut Shrimp

Ingredients

- 1/2 cup (about 2 1/8 oz.) all-purpose flour
- 1/2 teaspoons black pepper
- large eggs
- 2/3 cup unsweetened flaked coconut
- 1/3 cup panko (Japanese-style breadcrumbs)
- 12 ounces medium peeled, deveined raw shrimp, tail-on (about 24 shrimp)
- Cooking spray
- 1/2 teaspoon kosher salt
- 1/4 cup honey
- 1/4 cup lime juice 1 serrano chile, thinly sliced

- teaspoons chopped fresh cilantro (optional)

Preparation

1. Stir together flour and pepper in a shallow dish. Lightly beat eggs in a second shallow dish. Stir together coconut and panko in a third shallow dish. Holding each shrimp by the tail, dredge shrimp in flour mixture, making sure not to coat tail; shake off excess. Dip in egg, allowing any excess to drip off. Dredge in coconut mixture, pressing to adhere. Coat shrimp well with cooking spray.

2. Place half of the shrimp in air fryer basket, and cook at 400°F until golden, 6 to 8 minutes, turning shrimp over halfway through cooking. Season with 1/4 teaspoon of the salt. Repeat with remaining shrimp and salt.

3. While shrimp cook, whisk together honey, lime juice, and serrano chile in small bowl. Sprinkle shrimp with cilantro, if desired. Serve with sauce

Air-Fried Corn Dog Bites

Ingredients

- 2 uncured all-beef hot dogs
- 12 craft sticks or bamboo skewers
- 1/2 cup (about 2 1/8 oz.) all-purpose flour
- 2 large eggs, lightly beaten
- 1/2 cups finely crushed cornflakes cereal
- Cooking spray
- 8 teaspoons yellow mustard

Preparation

1. Slice each hot dog in half lengthwise. Cut each half into 3 equal pieces. Insert a craft stick or bamboo skewer into 1 end of each piece of hot dog.

2. Place flour in a shallow dish. Place lightly beaten eggs in a second shallow dish. Place crushed cornflakes in a third shallow dish. Dredge hot dogs in flour, shaking off excess. Dip in egg, allowing any excess to drip off. Dredge in cornflake crumbs, pressing to adhere.

3. Lightly coat air fryer basket with cooking spray. Place 6 corn dog bites in basket; lightly spray tops with cooking spray. Cook at 375°F until coating is golden brown and crunchy, 10 minutes, turning the corn dog bites over halfway through cooking. Repeat with remaining corn dog bites.

4. To serve, place 3 corn dog bites on each plate with 2 teaspoons mustard and serve immediately.

Crispy Toasted Sesame Tofu

Ingredients

- 2 (14-oz.) pkg. extra-firm tofu, drained and cut into 1-inch cubes
- Cooking spray
- 1/4 cup fresh orange juice (from 1 orange)
- 2 tablespoons lower-sodium soy sauce
- tablespoon plus 1 tsp. honey
- 1 tablespoon plus 1 tsp. toasted sesame oil
- 1 teaspoon rice vinegar
- 1/2 teaspoon

Preparation

1. Preheat oven 200°F.

2. Place tofu on a plate lined with several layers of paper towels; cover with additional paper towels and a second plate. Place a weight on top. Let stand 30 minutes. Coat tofu with cooking spray.

3. Place half of the tofu in single layer in air fryer basket, and cook at 375°F until crispy and golden brown, about 15 minutes, turning tofu cubes over halfway through cooking. Keep warm in preheated oven while cooking remaining tofu.

4. Meanwhile, whisk together orange juice, soy sauce, honey, sesame oil,

rice vinegar, and cornstarch in a small saucepan over high. Bring to a boil, whisking constantly, until sauce thickens, 2 to 3 minutes. Remove from heat; set aside.

5. Prepare rice according to package directions. Stir in salt.

6. Toss tofu with soy sauce mixture. Divide rice among 4 bowls; top with tofu. Sprinkle with scallions and sesame seeds.

Air-Fried Beet Chips

Ingredients

3 medium-size red beets (about 1 1/2 lb.), peeled and cut into 1/8-inch thick slices (about 3 cups slices)

2 teaspoons canola oil

3/4 teaspoon kosher salt

1/4 teaspoon black pepper

Preparation

- Toss sliced beets, oil, salt, and pepper in a large bowl.

- Place half of the beets in air fryer basket, and cook at 320°F until dry and crisp, 25 to 30 minutes, shaking the basket every 5 minutes. Repeat with remaining beets.

Air Fryer Veggie Quesadillas

Ingredients

- 4 (6-in.) sprouted whole-grain flour tortillas
- 4 ounces reduced-fat sharp Cheddar cheese, shredded (about 1 cup)
- cup sliced red bell pepper 1 cup sliced zucchini 1 cup no-salt-added canned black beans, drained and rinsed
- Cooking spray
- ounces plain 2% reduced-fat Greek yogurt
- 1 teaspoon lime zest plus 1 Tbsp. fresh juice (from 1 lime)
- 1/4 teaspoon ground cumin
- tablespoons chopped fresh cilantro
- 1/2 cup drained refrigerated pico de gallo

Preparation

1. Place tortillas on a work surface. Sprinkle 2 tablespoons shredded cheese over half of each tortilla. Top cheese on each tortilla with 1/4 cup each red pepper slices, zucchini slices, and black beans. Sprinkle evenly with remaining 1/2 cup cheese. Fold tortillas over to form half-moon shaped quesadillas. Lightly coat quesadillas with cooking spray, and secure with toothpicks.

2. Lightly spray air fryer basket with cooking spray. Carefully place 2 quesadillas in the basket, and cook at 400°F until tortillas are golden brown and slightly crispy, cheese is melted, and vegetables are slightly softened, 10 minutes, turning quesadillas over halfway through

cooking. Repeat with remaining quesadillas.

3. While quesadillas cook, stir together yogurt, lime zest, lime juice, and cumin in a small bowl. To serve, cut each quesadilla into wedges and sprinkle with cilantro. Serve each with 1 tablespoon cumin cream and 2 tablespoons pico de gallo.

Air-Fried Breakfast Bombs

Ingredients

- 3 center-cut bacon slices
- 3 large eggs, lightly beaten
- ounce 1/3-less-fat cream cheese, softened
- 1 tablespoon chopped fresh chives
- 4 ounces fresh prepared whole-wheat pizza dough
- Cooking spray

Preparation

1. Cook bacon in a medium skillet over medium until very crisp, about 10 minutes. Remove bacon from pan; crumble. Add eggs to bacon drippings in pan; cook, stirring often, until almost set but still loose, about 1 minute. Transfer eggs to a bowl; stir in cream cheese, chives, and crumbled bacon.

2. Divide dough into 4 equal pieces. Roll each piece on a lightly floured surface into a 5-inch circle. Place one-fourth of egg mixture in center of each dough circle. Brush outside edge of dough with water; wrap dough around egg mixture to form a purse, pinching together dough at the seams.

3. Place dough purses in single layer in air fryer basket; coat well with cooking spray. Cook at 350°F until golden brown, 5 to 6 minutes, checking after 4 minutes.

Air-Fried Curry Chickpeas

Ingredients

- (15-oz.) can no-salt-added chickpeas (garbanzo beans), drained and rinsed (about 1 1/2 cups)
- tablespoons red wine vinegar
- tablespoons olive oil
- 2 teaspoons curry powder
- 1/2 teaspoon ground turmeric
- 1/4 teaspoon ground coriander
- 1/4 teaspoon ground cumin
- 1/4 teaspoon plus 1/8 tsp. ground cinnamon
- 1/4 teaspoon kosher salt
- 1/2 teaspoon Aleppo pepper
- Thinly sliced fresh cilantro

Preparation

1. Gently smash chickpeas with your hands in a medium bowl (do not crush); discard chickpea skins.

2. Add vinegar and oil to chickpeas, and toss to coat. Add curry powder, turmeric, coriander, cumin, and cinnamon; stir gently to combine.

3. Place chickpeas in single layer in air fryer basket, and cook at 400°F until crispy, about 15 minutes, shaking chickpeas halfway through cooking.

4. Transfer chickpeas to a bowl. Sprinkle with salt, Aleppo pepper, and cilantro; toss to coat.

Air Fryer "Everything Bagel" Kale Chips

Ingredients

- 6 cups packed torn Lacinato kale leaves, stems and ribs removed
- tablespoon olive oil
- 1 teaspoon lower-sodium soy sauce
- 1 teaspoon white or black sesame seeds
- 1/2 teaspoon dried minced garlic
- 1/4 teaspoon poppy seeds

Preparation

1. Wash and completely dry kale leaves, and tear into 1 1/2-inch pieces. Toss together kale, olive oil, and soy sauce in a medium

bowl, rubbing the leaves gently to be sure they are well coated with mixture.

2. Place one-third of the kale leaves in air fryer basket, and cook at 375°F until crisp, 6 minutes, shaking basket halfway through cooking. Place kale chips on a baking sheet, and sprinkle evenly with sesame seeds, garlic, and poppy seeds while still hot. Repeat with remaining kale leaves.

Air Fry These Shrimp Spring Rolls With Sweet Chili Sauce

Ingredients

- 2 1/2 tablespoons sesame oil, divided
- 2 cups pre-shredded cabbage
- cup matchstick carrots
- 1 cup julienne-cut red bell pepper
- 4 ounces peeled, deveined raw shrimp, chopped
- 3/4 cup julienne-cut snow peas
- 1/4 cup chopped fresh cilantro
- 1 tablespoon fresh lime juice
- teaspoons fish sauce
- 1/4 teaspoon crushed red pepper
- 8 (8-inch-square) spring roll wrappers
- 1/2 cup sweet chili sauce

Preparation

1. Heat 1 1/2 teaspoons of the oil in large skillet over high until slightly smoking. Add cabbage, carrots, and bell pepper; cook, stirring constantly until lightly wilted, 1 to 1 1/2 minutes. Spread on a rimmed baking sheet; cool 5 minutes.

2. Place cabbage mixture, shrimp, snow peas, cilantro, lime juice, fish sauce, and crushed red pepper in a large bowl; toss to combine.

3. Place spring roll wrappers on work surface with 1 corner facing you. Spoon 1/4 cup filling in center of each spring roll wrapper, spreading from left to right into a 3-inch long strip. Fold bottom corner of each wrapper over filling, tucking tip of corner under filling. Fold left and right corners over filling. Lightly brush remaining corner with water; tightly roll

filled end toward remaining corner; gently press to seal. Brush spring rolls with remaining 2 tablespoons oil.

4. Place 4 spring rolls in air fryer basket, and cook at 390°F until golden, 6 to 7 minutes, turning spring rolls after 5 minutes. Repeat with remaining spring rolls. Serve with sweet chili sauce.

Spicy Zucchini Slices

Preparation Time: 10 minutes
Cooking Time: 6 minutes

Ingredients:	Nutritional value
1 teaspoon cornstarch	Calories 67
1 zucchini	Fat 2.4
½ teaspoon chili flakes	Protein 4.4
1 tablespoon flour	Carbohydrate 7.7
1 egg	
¼ teaspoon salt	

Directions:
1. Slice the zucchini and sprinkle with the chili flakes and salt. Whisk the egg into the bowl. Dip the zucchini slices into the whisked egg.

2. Combine cornstarch with the flour. Stir it. Coat the zucchini slices with the cornstarch mixture—Preheat the air fryer to 400 F.

3. Put the zucchini slices in the air fryer tray. Cook for 4 minutes, then flip the pieces to another side and cook for 2 minutes more. Serve the zucchini slices hot.

Cheddar Portobello Mushrooms

Preparation Time: 15 minutes
Cooking Time: 6 minutes

Ingredients:	Nutritional value
2 Portobello mushroom hats	Calories 376
2 slices Cheddar cheese	Fat 24.1
¼ cup panko breadcrumbs	Protein 25
½ teaspoon salt	Carb 14.6
½ teaspoon ground black pepper	
1 egg	
1 teaspoon oatmeal	
2 oz. bacon, chopped cooked	

Directions:
1. Whisk the egg into the bowl. Combine the ground black pepper, oatmeal, salt, and breadcrumbs in a separate bowl.

2. Dip the mushroom hats in the whisked egg. After this, coat the mushroom hats in the breadcrumb mixture.

3. Warm air fryer to 400 F. Place the mushrooms in the air fryer basket tray and cook for 3 minutes.

4. After this, put the chopped bacon and sliced cheese over the mushroom hats and cook the meal for 3 minutes. When the meal is cooked – let it chill gently.

Salty Lemon Artichokes

Preparation Time: 15 minutes
Cooking Time: 45 minutes

Ingredients:	Nutritional value
1 lemon	Calories 133
2 artichokes	Fat 5g
1 teaspoon kosher salt	Protein 6g
1 garlic head	Carb 21.7g
2 teaspoons olive oil	

Directions:

1. Cut off the edges of the artichokes. Cut the lemon into halves. Peel the garlic head and chop the garlic cloves roughly.

2. Then place the chopped garlic in the artichokes. Sprinkle the artichokes with olive oil and kosher salt. Then squeeze the lemon juice into the artichokes. Wrap the artichokes in the foil.

3. Preheat the air fryer to 330 F. Place the wrapped artichokes in the air fryer and cook for 45 minutes. When the artichokes are cooked – discard the foil and serve.

Cheddar Potato Gratin

Preparation Time: 15 minutes
Cooking Time: 20 minutes

Ingredients:	**Nutritional value**
2 potatoes, thinly sliced	Calories 353
1/3 cup half and half	Fat 16.6g
1 tablespoon oatmeal flour	Protein 15g
¼ teaspoon ground black pepper	Carb 37.2g
1 egg	
2 oz. Cheddar cheese	

Directions:

1. Preheat the air fryer to 365 F. Put the potato slices in the air fryer and cook them for 10 minutes.

Meanwhile, combine the half and half, oatmeal flour, and ground black pepper. Crack the egg

Breaded Air Fried Shrimp with Bang-Bang Sauce

Ingredients:	Nutritional value
3/4 cup whole wheat bread crumbs 4 cups raw shrimp, deveined, peeled 1 tsp ½ cup flour 1 tsp paprika chicken seasoning, to taste 2 tbsp. of one egg white kosher salt and pepper to taste Bang-Bang Sauce: ¼ cup sweet chili sauce 1/3 cup plain Greek yogurt 2 tbsp sriracha	Calories 229 Fat 10g Protein 22g Carb 13g

Preparation time: 10 minutes
Cooking time: 20 minutes

Directions:

1. Let the Air Fryer preheat to 400 degrees. Add the seasonings to shrimp and coat well. In three separate bowls, add flour, bread crumbs, and egg whites.

2. First coat the shrimp in flour, dab lightly in egg whites, then in the bread crumbs. With cooking oil, spray the shrimp.

3. Place the shrimps in an air fryer, cook for four minutes, turn the shrimp over, and cook for another four minutes. In a small bowl, mix all the bang-bang ingredients. Serve with micro green and bang-bang sauce.

Shrimp Egg Rolls

Preparation time: 20 minutes
Cooking time: 20 minutes

Ingredients:	**Nutritional value**
2-3 cloves of minced garlic 12-14 egg roll wrappers 2-3 cloves of minced garlic 4 cups raw shrimp, roughly chopped, peeled, and deveined 3 cups coleslaw mix 1 ½ tsp sesame oil 1 tbsp soy sauce 1 tsp fish sauce salt, pepper to taste ½ tsp grated ginger 2 green onions, chopped 1 cup water	Calories 228 Fat 11g Protein 20g Carb 11g

Directions:

1. In a skillet, add shrimp with garlic, kosher salt, and pepper, spray with cooking oil and sauté until shrimp is pink. Set it aside.
2. In a bowl, add coleslaw mix, cooked shrimp, green onions, fish sauce, soy sauce, sesame oil, and ginger. Mix well.
3. Add two tbsp of filling to each wrapper, seal tightly with water. With cooking oil, spray the air fryer basket. Put the egg rolls in a single layer in the basket. Spray with cooking oil.
4. Cook for 7 minutes at 400 degrees. Flip the rolls, then cook for 5 minutes more. Serve with a microgreen salad.

Chocolate Almond Butter Brownie

Preparation Time: 10 minutes

Cooking Time: 16 minutes

Ingredients:	Nutritional value
1 cup bananas, overripe	Calories 82
1/2 cup almond butter, melted	Fat 2g
1 scoop protein powder	Protein 7g
2 tbsp unsweetened cocoa powder	Carb 11g

Directions:

1. Warm air fryer to 325 F. Grease air fryer baking pan and set aside. Blend all fixings in a blender until smooth.

2. Pour batter into the prepared pan and place in the air fryer basket, and cook for 16 minutes. Serve and enjoy.

Parmesan Sweet Potato Casserole

Preparation Time: 15 minutes
Cooking Time: 35 minutes

Ingredients:	Nutritional value
2 sweet potatoes, peeled, chopped	Calories 93
½ yellow onion, sliced	Fat 1.8g
½ cup cream	Protein 1.8g
¼ cup spinach, chopped	Carb 20.3g
2 oz. Parmesan cheese, shredded	
½ teaspoon salt	
1 tomato, chopped	
1 teaspoon olive oil	

Directions:

1. Spray the air fryer tray with the olive oil. Then place on the layer of the chopped sweet potato. Add the layer of the sliced onion.

2. After this, sprinkle the sliced onion with the chopped spinach and tomatoes. Sprinkle the casserole with salt and shredded cheese. Pour cream.

3. Preheat the air fryer to 390 F. Cover the air fryer tray with the foil. Cook the casserole for 35 minutes. When the casserole is cooked – serve it.

Asparagus & Parmesan

Preparation Time: 10 minutes
Cooking Time: 6 minutes

Ingredients:	Nutritional value
1 teaspoon sesame oil	Calories 189
11 oz. asparagus	Fat 11.6g
1 teaspoon chicken stock	Protein 17.2g
½ teaspoon ground white pepper	Carb 7.9g
3 oz. Parmesan	

Directions:

1. Wash the asparagus and chop it roughly. Sprinkle the chopped asparagus with the chicken stock and ground white pepper.

2. Then sprinkle the vegetables with the sesame oil and shake them. Place the asparagus in the air fryer basket— Cook the vegetables for 4 minutes at 400 F.

3. Meanwhile, shred Parmesan cheese. When the time is over – shake the asparagus gently and sprinkle with the shredded cheese.

4. Cook the asparagus for 2 minutes more at 400 F. After this, transfer the cooked asparagus to the serving plates. Serve and taste it!

Thanks again for choosing this book, make sure to leave a short review on amazon if you enjoy it, I would really love to hear your thoughts.